Dear Reader,

Deeds, not words. You don't need seventeenth-century writer John Fletcher to tell you that the hot new bestseller you've just read on losing weight won't do you a bit of good if you don't put those 300 or so pages full of words into action.

The book you hold in your hands is the equivalent of a toolbox that will help you—no matter what diet you choose—rework your old way of eating into a new, healthier lifestyle. As everyone who has ever watched an exercise video while eating buttered popcorn in a recliner chair knows, you won't lose weight sitting on the sidelines. You have to get into the action, or your diet won't work.

How do you do this? Writing and keeping your medical history in one easy-to-find place, maintaining a food diary for a long enough time so that you can really see where your diet is succeeding (or going bust), and integrating exercise into your daily life are just three ways to turn a diet book's words into a smaller waist, stronger muscles, and a healthier heart.

From this book you'll learn what to expect from your diet from the first euphoric days of weight loss to the steady, smaller losses of the long haul. You'll learn how to resist the temptations of restaurants and holidays and how to handle the psychological pitfalls inherent in losing weight. You'll learn some danger points and how to avoid them. You'll also have a handy nutritional guide to more than 1,000 foods—an essential for any diet.

In short, this book is the best friend who's always on call to encourage you, nudge you, or enlighten you when you need that small, still voice to keep you on track.

The rewards? Getting into your "thin" jeans and having them be loose, hearing your doctor say your heart sounds great, and acquiring the confidence to stand up and take your place in life.

Happy dieting! Losing weight is within reach, and you're holding the best guidebook there is to get you to your goal.

Shirley Mathews

Jyni Holland, M.S., R.D.

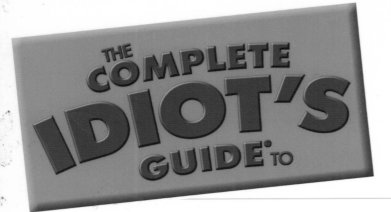

THE COMPLETE IDIOT'S GUIDE TO

Keep track of your low-carb, low-cal, low-fat diet and exercise program. It's easy with this handy tracker!

Weight Loss

TRACKER

♦ **The tools you need** to reach your weight-loss goals

♦ **Complete nutrition tables** on over 2000 foods

♦ **The perfect companion** to your favorite diet and exercise books

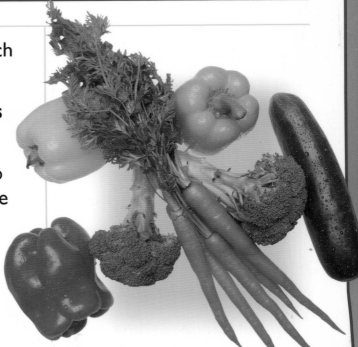

Shirley Mathews and
Jyni Holland, M.S., R.D.

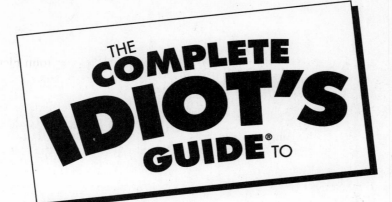

Weight Loss
Tracker

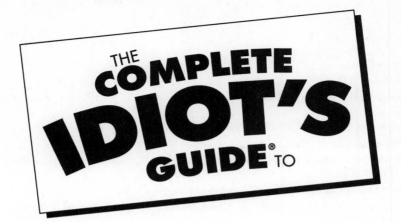

THE COMPLETE IDIOT'S GUIDE® TO

Weight Loss Tracker

by Shirley Mathews and
Jyni Holland, M.S., R.D.

ALPHA

A member of Penguin Group (USA) Inc.

ALPHA BOOKS

Published by the Penguin Group

Penguin Group (USA) Inc., 375 Hudson Street, New York, New York 10014, U.S.A.

Penguin Group (Canada), 10 Alcorn Avenue, Toronto, Ontario, Canada M4V 3B2 (a division of Pearson Penguin Canada Inc.)

Penguin Books Ltd, 80 Strand, London WC2R 0RL, England

Penguin Ireland, 25 St Stephen's Green, Dublin 2, Ireland (a division of Penguin Books Ltd)

Penguin Group (Australia), 250 Camberwell Road, Camberwell, Victoria 3124, Australia (a division of Pearson Australia Group Pty Ltd)

Penguin Books India Pvt Ltd, 11 Community Centre, Panchsheel Park, New Delhi—110 017, India

Penguin Group (NZ), cnr Airborne and Rosedale Roads, Albany, Auckland 1310, New Zealand (a division of Pearson New Zealand Ltd)

Penguin Books (South Africa) (Pty) Ltd, 24 Sturdee Avenue, Rosebank, Johannesburg 2196, South Africa

Penguin Books Ltd, Registered Offices: 80 Strand, London WC2R 0RL, England

Most Alpha books are available at special quantity discounts for bulk purchases for sales promotions, premiums, fundraising, or educational use. Special books, or book excerpts, can also be created to fit specific needs.

For details, write: Special Markets, Alpha Books, 375 Hudson Street, New York, NY 10014.

Publisher: *Marie Butler-Knight*
Product Manager: *Phil Kitchel*
Senior Managing Editor: *Jennifer Bowles*
Senior Acquisitions Editor: *Mike Sanders*
Development Editor: *Michael Koch*

Senior Production Editor: *Billy Fields*
Copy Editor: *Tricia Liebig*
Cover/Book Designer: *Trina Wurst*
Indexer: *Angie Bess*
Layout: *Rebecca Harmon*

To my mother and father and to my infinitely wonderful husband, Owen. S.M.
To my mother, Helen Holland. J.H.

Contents at a Glance

List of Tables

List of Figures

Contents

Introduction

Whether you're counting calories; adding up points or exchanges; doing the balancing act with carbohydrates, protein, and fat; or trying to lose pounds some other way, there's one thread that connects you to every other dieter: You have to keep on your diet if you want to lose weight.

This book will keep you aimed in the right direction and alert you when you're straying off into old, fattening habits. It will also be a valuable resource in an emergency; you'll have all your medical and drug information, your family history, and much more collected within the covers of this book. Never hunt through closets, drawers, and files looking for half-forgotten phone numbers, drug doses, or doctors' names again!

You'll also find out the easiest (and cheapest) way to start getting yourself into shape—and how to stay in shape throughout your life. You'll learn that certain drugs and foods can throw up roadblocks to prevent your weight loss, and we tell you the pros and cons of breaking through these obstacles.

Most important, we give you the detailed nutritional breakdown of more than 1,000 foods in a handy table at the back of this book, so you can gauge exactly what nutrients you need and the foods that contain them. Need to know how many net carbs are in ketchup? Look it up here. Need to know how many calories are in a hamburger? This table's got all this and much, much more. Everything you need to lose weight is within these pages.

How This Book Is Organized

This book has six chapters.

Chapter 1 creates a snapshot of how your health is right now, taking into account the conditions blood relatives have that may affect your own health. You'll also create a profile of what treatments and drugs you are taking—an invaluable tool if you ever have an emergency. You'll find out how to calculate how much you should weigh, and you'll fill in a food diary that will give you an in-depth look at what your present diet is like. All these tools will help you springboard into your new thinner lifestyle.

Chapter 2 guides you through the undiscovered territory of the first few weeks of your new diet. We arm you with knowledge, so side effects won't take you by surprise. You can read tips on how to beat the diet blues and break a binge. Further, this chapter simply lays out how to pick out and buy the most healthful meats, fruits, and vegetables; how to store them; and how to tell when you should throw them away! You will master the fine art of decoding food labels—hidden sugars and fats will be annoyances of the past.

Chapter 3 is the bridge between the safety of your own kitchen and the relative danger of the rest of the world. Food is the universal language of weddings and other events, and restaurants can hold your diet hostage to everything forbidden. Find out how to skirt the landmines and breeze through these temptations by defusing the crises before they even come up. Also discover how being tired or stressed can trip up even the most well-laid out of diet plans.

Chapter 4 shows you that easy-does-it when it comes to exercise is the best possible plan. Walking is basic, but you'll also discover that the two easiest exercises—shallow squats and graduated pushups—can lead to a lifetime of toned muscles and controlled weight. Finally, we'll show you a simple way to figure out how fast your metabolism is and what your basic caloric requirements are.

Chapter 5 addresses what few books ever touch on: What happens when you start to lose weight, and you go from being invisible to the center of attention. Fear, intimidation, and confusion can sabotage your weight loss. Read here how you can redirect those feelings and rediscover your inspiration to lose.

Chapter 6 outlines what can flat line your diet. Alcohol and tobacco may have effects you don't suspect that can prevent weight loss. And chocolate and caffeine? Read here about how they can waylay even the most dedicated of dieters. Also, prescription and over-the-counter drugs may also affect your weight loss, but the dangers of altering your medications can be profound. We detail some consequences here.

The appendixes at the end of this book provide tools and information that help you master your diet regimen. We start you off with several Daily Journal forms where you can keep track of not only your food intake, but also your exercise and other diet essentials. When you need more, just photocopy the basic blank form and compile your own diet notebook. You can graph your weight in Appendix B to get a long-term visual sense of how you're doing and track whether your diet is stalling. You can also browse through the list of interactive websites, a glossary, and, most importantly the Nutritive Table of Foods, Appendix C.

Appendix C serves up a table that provides an exhaustive list of more than 1,000 foods, ranging from apples and beer to potatoes and breakfast cereals. Never again wonder how much protein, fat, carbohydrates, or calories a food contains! You can calculate your daily diet and set a goal for yourself each day.

A la Carte

The tips, alerts, definitions, and facts highlighted on each page are the signposts on your road to a healthy and fit body.

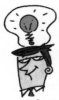

Tips to Use _____

Follow these words of wisdom and common sense, and you won't go wrong on your diet.

These facts shine a revealing light on general aspects of dieting and provide interesting tidbits for all dieters.

What's That Mean? _____

Unfamiliar terms and words are demystified in these helpful boxes.

Diet Alert _____

These warnings are geared to try to head you off from any danger that may lie in your path.

Acknowledgments

Teamwork takes on a new meaning when you start writing a book, and I owe so much to so many. Jeannette and Richard Mathews taught me I could do anything I set my mind to, and you hold the proof of that in your hands. Thanks also to the Pettigrew Drive Research S.W.A.T. Team; without Neal and Peggy Easom and Owen O'Neill, I never would have made my deadlines. Many thanks to my agent, Marilyn Allen, for steering this project my way, and a big tip of the hat to my patient and kind editor, Mike Sanders. Lastly, Colette Bouchez has been an inspiration and a true friend, and she's always been ready to put the cool hand to the fevered forehead. Deep thanks to all of you!

—Shirley Mathews

I would like to thank my mother, Helen Holland, for her love and support and for being my constant source of strength; my sister Tracey Holland, who is always there for me; Lyne Marcellus, fellow dietitian and study mate. Lyne, I could not have done this without you. I also thank my dear friends Lori Anne Borries and Joanne Bosch for their support and concern while I was in the master's program; Anne Caron for being the amazing friend and woman that you are; Lisa Sasson and Gail Torres for believing in me; Geraline Adames for her encouragement; and my sister Kim Santiago for always being proud of me and my work. Finally, I thank any and all who have provided love, support, and encouragement during this journey.

—Jyni Holland, M.S., R.D.

Trademarks

All terms mentioned in this book that are known to be or are suspected of being trademarks or service marks have been appropriately capitalized. Alpha Books and Penguin Group (USA) Inc. cannot attest to the accuracy of this information. Use of a term in this book should not be regarded as affecting the validity of any trademark or service mark.

Sworn to Lose

In This Chapter

- Establishing your health baseline
- Compiling a family, medicine, and health history
- Figuring out your weight-loss goals
- Comparing your health to the "norms"
- Taking stock of your present diet

Your diet book is in front of you. You've skimmed the charts and graphs, you've read the blurbs and promises, and now you're ready to start losing weight in earnest.

But wait.

A little care and planning in the beginning will pay off in the long run. Also, taking some time now to document what your family health history is, what your own health is like now, and the physical details of your body is not only good for those late-in-the-diet attaboys that you'll need to steel your resolve, but might also make a difference in how you approach your diet or what you might have to ask your doctor.

In this chapter you'll establish where your baseline is in many aspects of your life. By filling in forms and examining the various tables in this section, you'll be able to have at your fingertips such vital information as doctor contacts, medications and doses, possible problems between some common over-the-counter drugs and your new regimen, your body measurements and frame type, and many other evaluators.

This chapter also discusses some tests your doctor might want you to take before you start your diet, talks about what your goals and expectations are, and gives you a few cautionary words to prepare you for surprises that may appear as your excess pounds disappear.

You'll keep a food diary for a week for a graphic look at where your diet is right now. Filling in this diary will also keep you grounded as you progress in your diet. Nothing will feel better for you than comparing a food diary a few months from now to the one you are about to fill out. The most shocking—and satisfying—thing in this experience may be realizing how poorly you were eating before you began your diet.

Above all, this book is dedicated to helping you make your diet a positive, safe, and successful experience. The medical "snapshot" of your family and other tools in this chapter will help lay the groundwork to start your weight-loss plan of action.

Taking Stock

Before looking to the future, however, you should look to the past. The first thing to do is to get your medical history down in black and white.

Having a medical inventory of yourself is one of the most useful references you can create. As far as your health goes, it will tell you where you came from, it might provide clues as to where you are headed, and will tell you if you should be prepared for any stumbling blocks along the way.

Charting Your Family's Health History

The following Family History form is designed to provide an at-a-glance look of your family's longevity and what might affect your own efforts at weight loss. Not every column will apply. For instance, you will only be able to fill in your own body type and whether you are a smoker on your own line. If some relatives listed are still living, fill in what applies; it will still give you a general profile of your family.

Family History

Relative	Still Living?	Body Type*	Age at Death	Cause of Death	Smoker (Y or N)
Mother	No	Obese	67	card	N
Father	No	O.W→Thin	91	resp	N
Sister	No	Thin	65	alzh	N
Sister	Yes	Norm			N
Brother	Yes	OW			N
Brother					
Aunts	Yes	Norm			N
Aunts	yes	Thin			N
Uncles	No	Norm		UK	UK
Uncles	No	Obese		UK	UK
Mother's Father	No	OW → Norm	78	resp	N
Mother's Mother	No	Obese → Norm	82	heart	N
Father's Father	No	UK	UK	UK	UK
Father's Mother	No	OW	60's	UK	N
You	N/A	Obese			
Other Blood Relatives					

*Use thin, normal, overweight, or obese

Going hand-in-hand with a family profile like the one in the Family History form is a history of disease among your blood relatives. Many diseases are linked to heredity; other diseases seem to spring from a common trigger, such as heart disease and obesity. Fill out the My Health Heredity form as completely as you can. Ask parents and siblings, if possible, if they know more about diseases in your family. After you have all the results laid out in one place, you might be surprised to see some trends in your family.

Once you're finished making notes and checking off what applies, take a hard look at everyone whose genes you carry. Is there a pattern? Did all the men in your family die young of heart disease? Did all the women have breast cancer? Are there recurring illnesses or weight issues on either—or both—sides of the family? These are trends you and your doctor need to know.

Cancer may seem to be a surprising addition to this table, but certain types of cancer do seem to have a definite relationship to obesity. What's the difference between overweight and obese? If you're 5 feet 5 inches tall and weigh 150 pounds, you're overweight. If you're the same height and weigh 180 pounds, you're at the threshold of obesity.

A weight/cancer cause-and-effect is not clear-cut because in obese people, there is usually a host of other factors that also contribute to the disease. For example, researchers in colon cancer don't know if the disease is caused by the obesity itself or a diet that generally skimps on fruits and vegetables and goes heavy on high-fat, high-calorie foods.

Again, you may not have all the information to fill in the blanks, but don't beat yourself up. This is a tool to help you, not a test you pass or fail. Some fuzziness in the details is normal.

My Health Heredity

Condition	You	Mother	Father	Grand-parents	Siblings	Other Blood Relatives
Allergies	✓		✓		✓	
Arthritis				✓		
Asthma						
Cancer			✓		✓	
Bladder						
Breast					✓	
Colon						
Gallbladder						
Kidney						
Prostate			✓		✓	
Uterus						
Circulation Problems				✓		
Depression	✓	✓				
Diabetes						
Gallbladder						
Heart Disease		✓	✓	✓		
High Blood Pressure		✓	✓	✓		
High Cholesterol	✓	✓	✓		✓	
Kidney						
Obesity	✓	✓		✓		
Osteoporosis						
Sleep Problems	✓		✓			
Stroke						
Thyroid Problems	✓	✓			✓	
Other						
Comments						

Measuring Up

Look around you. If you're standing in line at the supermarket, watching a movie at a theater, or eating in a restaurant, more than 6 out of 10 of all the people you see are overweight. Nearly one out of every three of those overweight people is obese. How do you tell where you fit in? One way of calculating your ideal weight is to do it as a relationship between your height and weight. This is called the *Body Mass Index* (*BMI*) and is a good indication of how much fat is on your body.

The following table shows the ranges of BMI and what they mean.

How do you find where you are in this list? Take a look at the following BMI chart. Find your height, in inches, on the left side, then following that row across, find your weight within the chart. At the top of the column with your weight is your BMI number. Find where that number fits into the BMI chart, and you'll have a better idea of where you're starting from.

What's That Mean?

Body Mass Index (BMI) is a relationship between weight and height that measures fat in the body. It is figured by dividing your weight in pounds by the square of your height in inches and then multiplying that number by 703.

Note that BMI is a good indication, but it's not the entire story. Women naturally have more body fat than men, and people who are heavily muscled will come in with a high BMI that doesn't reflect their true body fat. Also, older people who have lost muscle mass may end up with a too-low BMI.

BMI Ranges

Weight	BMI
Underweight	less than 18.5
Normal weight	18.5 to 24.9
Overweight	25 to 29.9
Obese	30 or more

BMI Chart

Body Mass Index Table																																			
	Normal						Overweight					Obese										Extreme Obesity													
BMI	19	20	21	22	23	24	25	26	27	28	29	30	31	32	33	34	35	36	37	38	39	40	41	42	43	44	45	46	47	48	49	50	51	52	53	54
Height (inches)	Body Weight (pounds)																																			
58	91	96	100	105	110	115	119	124	129	134	138	143	148	153	158	162	167	172	177	181	186	191	196	201	205	210	215	220	224	229	234	239	244	248	253	258
59	94	99	104	109	114	119	124	128	133	138	143	148	153	158	163	168	173	178	183	188	193	198	203	208	212	217	222	227	232	237	242	247	252	257	262	267
60	97	102	107	112	118	123	128	133	138	143	148	153	158	163	168	174	179	184	189	194	199	204	209	215	220	225	230	235	240	245	250	255	261	266	271	276
61	100	106	111	116	122	127	132	137	143	148	153	158	164	169	174	180	185	190	195	201	206	211	217	222	227	232	238	243	248	254	259	264	269	275	280	285
62	104	109	115	120	126	131	136	142	147	153	158	164	169	175	180	186	191	196	202	207	213	218	224	229	235	240	246	251	256	262	267	273	278	284	289	295
63	107	113	118	124	130	135	141	146	152	158	163	169	175	180	186	191	197	203	208	214	220	225	231	237	242	248	254	259	265	270	278	282	287	293	299	304
64	110	116	122	128	134	140	145	151	157	163	169	174	180	186	192	197	204	209	215	221	227	232	238	244	250	256	262	267	273	279	285	291	296	302	308	314
65	114	120	126	132	138	144	150	156	162	168	174	180	186	192	198	204	210	216	222	228	234	240	246	252	258	264	270	276	282	288	294	300	306	312	318	324
66	118	124	130	136	142	148	155	161	167	173	179	186	192	198	204	210	216	223	229	235	241	247	253	260	266	272	278	284	291	297	303	309	315	322	328	334
67	121	127	134	140	146	153	159	166	172	178	185	191	198	204	211	217	223	230	236	242	249	255	261	268	274	280	287	293	299	306	312	319	325	331	338	344
68	125	131	138	144	151	158	164	171	177	184	190	197	203	210	216	223	230	236	243	249	256	262	269	276	282	289	295	302	308	315	322	328	335	341	348	354
69	128	135	142	149	155	162	169	176	182	189	196	203	209	216	223	230	236	243	250	257	263	270	277	284	291	297	304	311	318	324	331	338	345	351	358	365
70	132	139	146	153	160	167	174	181	188	195	202	209	216	222	229	236	243	250	257	264	271	278	285	292	299	306	313	320	327	334	341	348	355	362	369	376
71	136	143	150	157	165	172	179	186	193	200	208	215	222	229	236	243	250	257	265	272	279	286	293	301	308	315	322	329	338	343	351	358	365	372	379	386
72	140	147	154	162	169	177	184	191	199	206	213	221	228	235	242	250	258	265	272	279	287	294	302	309	316	324	331	338	346	353	361	368	375	383	390	397
73	144	151	159	166	174	182	189	197	204	212	219	227	235	242	250	257	265	272	280	288	295	302	310	318	325	333	340	348	355	363	371	378	386	393	401	408
74	148	155	163	171	179	186	194	202	210	218	225	233	241	249	256	264	272	280	287	295	303	311	319	326	334	342	350	358	365	373	381	389	396	404	412	420
75	152	160	168	176	184	192	200	208	216	224	232	240	248	256	264	272	279	287	295	303	311	319	327	335	343	351	359	367	375	383	391	399	407	415	423	431
76	156	164	172	180	189	197	205	213	221	230	238	246	254	263	271	279	287	295	304	312	320	328	336	344	353	361	369	377	385	394	402	410	418	426	435	443

Source: Adapted from *Clinical Guidelines on the Identification, Evaluation, and Treatment of Overweight and Obesity in Adults: The Evidence Report*.

Your BMI is a good indication of how much body fat you have.

(Courtesy of the National Heart, Lung, and Blood Institute's Clinical Guidelines on the Identification, Evaluation, and Treatment of Overweight and Obesity in Adults: The Evidence Report)

Listening to Your Heart Beat

Fat, blood, and your organs in general are all important, but don't forget about the engine that keeps the rest of your body moving: your heart.

A good indication as to where you are physically is how many times per minute your heart has to beat.

Check This Out

The heartbeat's normal range when resting is 60 to 100 beats per minute.

How do you figure this out? Put the tips of your index and middle fingers against the inside of the opposite wrist just below the mound at the base of your thumb. Count how many times your heart beats in 10 seconds and multiply by six. That will give you your heart rate per minute.

Every diet calls for exercise to one extent or another. As you exercise, your heart should, over time, become more efficient, and you should see your pulse slow. As you fill out the daily journal in Appendix A, make sure you keep track of the progress your heart is making, as well as the progress your entire body is making.

Charting Your Waist-to-Hip Ratio

Speaking of your body's progress—the easiest meaningful measurement you can take is that of your waist. For instance, a man with a waist size greater than 40 inches or a woman with a waist size greater than 35 inches are both at risk for heart disease, diabetes, high blood pressure, and other diseases.

CAUTION

Diet Alert

Waist measurement is not a foolproof indication of how much abdominal fat you are carrying. People who are short (under 5 feet tall) or people who are obese (a BMI of 35 or more) won't have waist measurements that apply to this general statement.

In fact, a good way of evaluating how your waist relates to other measurements and what this may mean for your health is by seeing what your *waist-to-hip ratio (WHR)* is. Fill in the blanks in the following form, and keep the results handy. In the coming weeks and months, you'll be able to see how this ratio changes as you lose weight and get into better shape.

Don't be put off by the math in this exercise; it's easy. Plus, this ratio will give you a good idea of how much you are at risk for such chronic diseases as diabetes and heart disease.

Find your waist-to-hip ratio by dividing your waist measurement by your hip measurement in the formula below. Simply fill in the blanks and do the math.

My Waist-to-Hip Ratio

_____ (waist measurement, in inches)

÷ _____ (hip measurement)

= _____ my WTH ratio

What's risky: A ratio of 1.0 or higher puts you in the danger zone for ailments connected with being overweight.

What's safe: For men, a ratio of 0.90 or less; for women, a ratio of 0.80 or less.

The Naked Truth About Your Body

After taking stock of your family's health history, you'll want to take stock of yourself—and keep taking this personal inventory as your diet continues. Many people find it helpful to make a copy of the various forms you'll be filling out and make your own notebook, so all your information is in one single place. Even after you've finished reading this book, it can still be a resource for you.

To begin, take a Polaroid, a digital image, or a good old-fashioned film photo of yourself and attach it to the form that follows. You'll be given more forms to complement your daily journal in Appendix A, but those forms will contain mostly information that changes from day to day. The first form is your jumping-off point, containing permanent as well as changeable information. This is the profile of yourself before you actually start your diet, and you'll have it as a reference if you ever need a boost to keep on your plan.

Tips to Use _____

It's best that you wear a bathing suit or some other costume that reveals your body in the photo. This way you can better tell over time how your body is changing. Too many clothes at this point will only hide your triumph down the line. After you've chosen your clothing for the photo, keep it handy and wear it when you want to take another reference photo. Nothing beats a picture for telling you the truth about how well you're doing.

Not all these measurements are essential—for instance, that of the upper arm—but some diets encourage taking even these measurements; they will help you see if one part of your body is losing inches faster than other parts.

Tips to Use _____

Having a set of "weigh-in" clothes helps because if the scale reading fluctuates, you need to be sure it is not due to different clothing than what you wore at the previous weigh-in.

Your height, as measured when you are in bare feet, will not change, so have that number handy. Also, you should always weigh yourself at the same time. Keep in mind, also, that most people are lightest at the beginning of the day before they've eaten or drunk anything.

Where does your weight fall in the following chart? The further to the right you are in this chart, the less healthy your weight is and the more prone you will be to overweight diseases, such as diabetes and heart disease.

Healthy Weight Chart.

(Source: Report of the Dietary Guidelines Advisory Committee on the Dietary Guidelines for Americans, 1995)

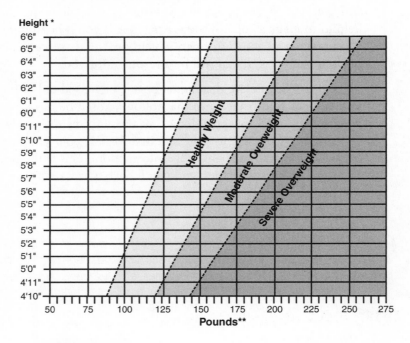

* Without shoes.
** Without clothes. The higher weights apply to people with more muscle and bone, such as many men.

Writing down your blood pressure and your blood cholesterol levels is another facet of charting your progress. Going on a diet commonly lowers both blood pressure and cholesterol. You'll want to keep track of both of these measurements; readings that spike or are too low could mean underlying problems you'll need to discuss with your doctor.

Your Blood Pressure

Blood pressure is the amount of force your blood exerts on your artery walls as it flows through your body. Although people may vary somewhat as to what constitutes "normal" for them, the National Heart, Lung, and Blood Institute considers the numbers in the following table a way to break down into optimal, normal, high-normal, and hypertensive (clinically speaking, high blood pressure).

Blood Pressure Readings

Optimal	Normal	High-Normal	Hypertensive
<120/80	<130/85	130–139/85–89	>140/90

The first number is the *systolic* reading (when the heart beats) and the second number is the *diastolic* reading (when the heart rests between beats).

What's That Mean?

Systolic is the top of the two numbers that measure blood pressure. This reflects the highest blood pressure reached as the blood is pumped out of the heart.

Diastolic is the bottom of the two blood pressure numbers. It reflects the blood's pressure when the heart is at rest between beats.

Your Moody Benchmarks

Your general mood—the way you move emotionally through each day—is not only a reflection of how you feel about yourself, but is also an indication as to how life is treating you. As you lose weight, look for these signposts to change.

Stresses you encounter virtually every day take a toll on you, both in your health and in your determination to succeed in your diet. Pinpointing these stresses will help you figure out solutions for dealing with them, and putting your solution down on paper is a major step toward putting the solution into action. The last item on this form is an inventory of the situations that may trigger a binge or other eating spree that might derail your diet. Knowing what they are can help you plan ahead for these potential triggers and disarm them before they blow your diet.

My Benchmarks

Name: _____

Today's date: _____

Height: _____

Weight: _____

Time I weighed myself: _____

What I was wearing: _____

Goal weight: _____

Other measurements: _____

  Waist: _____

  Hips: _____

  Chest: _____

  Upper arm: _____

  Thigh: _____

Date I started my diet: _____

Date photo was taken: _____

Blood pressure: _____

Blood type: _____

Total blood cholesterol: HDL ("good") LDL ("bad")

General mood (check all that apply):
❑ Happy ❑ Hopeful ❑ Determined ❑ Frustrated ❑ Angry ❑ Disappointed
❑ Sad ❑ Depressed ❑ Discouraged ❑ Tired ❑ Sleepy

Daily stresses (check all that apply):

❑ Ill child	❑ Child behavior	❑ Other child care issues	❑ Marital problems
❑ Family problems	❑ Job	❑ Boss	❑ Long hours
❑ Commute	❑ Cooking	❑ Cleaning	❑ Other housework
❑ Bereavement	❑ Ill	❑ Allergies active	❑ Other _____

One daily stress I will cope with better:

_____

How will I accomplish this?

_____

_____

Situations that trigger poor eating:
❑ Birthdays and other celebrations ❑ Holidays ❑ Restaurant dining ❑ Stressful
events or people (what or who are they?) _____

A Look in the Medicine Cabinet

The list of potential problems here is long, and consequences range from the potentially dangerous—taking insulin drugs if you're on an insulin-lowering diet (like a low-carb one, for instance)—to the merely irksome (sugar-laden cough drops, for example).

Don't forget that the most innocent-seeming over-the-counter drugs like aspirin and antacids must be taken into consideration because they may be at odds with your diet. Also, don't forget to account for any herbal remedies you may be taking; they might be harmless, but, then again, they might set the stage for a reaction you're not prepared for, such as jitteriness or nausea. At the very least, many drugs and herbals could simply make your weight loss stall, and this is a fact you want to be aware of. We'll talk more about stalls and plateaus in Chapter 2, but you should be alerted to the fact that medications may play a part in these frustrating episodes.

Filling in the Medication Inventory form that follows will help you keep track of what you are taking, the dosage, and if anything changes over time. Fill in the boxes with all the information about the medications and remedies you take. The words in italics are examples.

CAUTION   **Diet Alert** _____

The makers of Tylenol warn that you shouldn't take more than one over-the-counter drug that contains the same active ingredient unless your doctor or other health care professional okays it. How do you find the active ingredient? Look on the drug's label—usually there is a Drug Facts notice on the container. The first ingredient listed is the active ingredient.

Medication Inventory

Name: _____   Date: _____

Emergency contact/phone: _____

Primary care doctor/phone: _____

Drug allergies: _____

Reaction experienced: _____

Prescription Drugs

Brand Name	Generic Name	Dosage	Frequency	Reactions
Diabeta	Glyburide	1.25mg	1X a day	Sleepy

Over-the-Counter Drugs

Brand Name	Generic Name	Dosage	Frequency	Reactions
Tylenol	Acetaminophen	2 caplets	2X a week	None

Herbals

Brand Name	Technical Name	Dosage	Frequency	Reactions
St. John's Wort	Hypericum Perforatum	½ cup tea	3X a week	None

Vitamins and Supplements

Brand Name	Type	Dosage	Frequency	Reactions
One-A-Day	Calcium-Plus	W/500 mg of calcium	1X a week	None

Make sure that every doctor and specialist you are seeing has a copy of your Medication Inventory. This will help them adjust dosages, if needed, change medications safely, and keep from prescribing a drug that reacts with another drug you are taking.

Check This Out

If you want to start a low-carb diet and are on any medication that affects your blood sugar, liver, or kidney function, before you begin your diet, be sure that your doctor knows you are going on this type of regimen.

Also, eliminating food that raises insulin means that your body's insulin levels will lower. If you are a diabetic and are on medication for this disease, a low-carb diet might cause your insulin levels to lower so much that you may have a reaction to—or even overdose on—your medication. Talk to your doctor before starting a low-carb diet.

Diuretics

Even if your doctor has prescribed a diuretic for you, you should be aware that you may need to adjust your water drinking habits when you start your diet. This is especially true if you're starting a low-carb diet, which is naturally diuretic. All diets emphasize the importance of drinking water. If you don't take in enough water, you'll get dehydrated. Because the main reason people take a diuretic is to flush water from the system, you'll have to watch yourself closely to make sure you're not getting dehydrated.

Diet Alert

If your doctor has prescribed diuretics, don't decide by yourself to stop them. Talk to your doctor first before making any changes in your medications.

Another reason for drinking enough water is that your body, if dehydrated, may sometimes mistake thirst for hunger, triggering an eating binge. If you drink enough fluids, your body can't make this mistake, and you can keep to your diet more easily.

Over-the-Counter Medications

Many drugs are used so commonly and to such a large degree that it's easy to forget that they're really drugs. Don't make that mistake.

Check This Out

Some low-carb experts suggest you try to eliminate the unnecessary and optional minor medications from your life for at least a couple of weeks. At the end of that time, you'll have a better handle on whether you need them at all.

If you are taking drugs like cough drops (yes, they're drugs), cough syrups, antacids, antihistamines, aspirin and other anti-inflammatory drugs, throat soothers, stool softeners, or other such remedies for minor ailments, you should be aware that they may raise your insulin levels, thereby increasing your food cravings and throwing a wrench in your weight loss.

Again, if your doctor has recommended that you take a certain medication, even if it is over-the-counter, don't stop it without consulting with him or her first.

Tests Your Doctor May Want You to Take

If you have already taken the Chem-20 blood test (similar tests go by other names, but they all test *lipids* and organ function), that may be as much as you need to speed you along your way.

But your doctor may feel other tests are needed just to cover all the bases. What are the possible tests?

- **Blood pressure test.** Having this checked is so basic and routine during a doctor's visit that it's easy to forget about it. Make sure you ask your doctor to supply you with the results of your test.

- **Glucose tolerance test** (also called the oral *glucose* tolerance test). This test measures how well your body metabolizes glucose, the sugar the body uses for energy, and is usually done to see if the patient is likely to have diabetes. How is it usually done? You fast for 12 hours before the test. You then drink a solution with a set amount of glucose in it. Blood is drawn before the test and at various intervals after you drink the solution for up to three hours or so. Comparing the blood glucose levels in the samples will tell the doctor if you have a problem. What's considered normal— a reading of less than 140 mg/dL after two hours.

- **Thyroid test.** Your thyroid regulates your *metabolism*, and if it is working too slowly, you won't lose weight as quickly

What's That Mean?

Lipids are fatty substances in the blood that are sources of fuel and are easily stored by the body.

Glucose is the main source of your body's energy, and it is made from carbohydrates in food and transported through the body in the bloodstream.

What's That Mean?

Metabolism is everything your body does, chemically and physically, to keep growing and working. This has to do with the breaking down and building up of complex substances in the body. Breaking them down releases energy so that other complex substances, such as tissue and muscles, can be created.

as you'd like. If it is abnormally hard for you to lose weight, if you have high cholesterol, no energy, or retain fluid, your doctor may suggest testing this gland. If you have ever wondered why it is so hard to peel off those pounds once you reach a certain age, one of the many reasons is probably because your thyroid has naturally slowed production of its hormone.

If you're a woman, menopause—in both the "before" and "during" phases—may play havoc with your estrogen and throw off your thyroid, as well. If your doctor suspects an underactive thyroid, he or she might suggest tests that evaluate how well the gland is working and interacting with various other hormones and body chemicals. The test itself? You have some blood drawn. That's it.

Between keeping track of all the medicines, tests, measurements, and all the rest of the minutiae of your health may be a chore for you, and it may be even more complex for your doctors, especially if you are being treated by specialists. You'll want to keep everyone on the same page, and this book can help you do that.

Your Health Contact Sheet

It's always helpful to keep all your doctors apprised of what's going on. Filling out the Keeping Your Doctors on Track form with the names and contact numbers of all your doctors will not only help you, but it will also help them. Make copies of this form, and give one to each of your doctors. The more your health care providers know about what drugs you are getting and what other doctors are prescribing for treatment, the better able they will be to coordinate your care.

Also, having handy a form like this—one that includes your health insurance information—is invaluable in an emergency. Make sure your family members know where you keep this book or, if you are compiling your forms in one notebook, tell people where you have your information.

Keeping Your Doctors on Track

My Name: _____

Address: _____

City: _____ State: _____ ZIP: _____

Home phone: _____

Work phone: _____

Mobile phone: _____

Health insurance carrier: _____

Group, policy, or other insurance numbers: _____

Primary care doctor: _____

Office phone: _____

Nutritionist: _____

Office phone: _____

Specialist: _____

Office phone: _____

Specialist: _____

Office phone: _____

Specialist: _____

Office phone: _____

Your Weight-Loss Goals

Here's the first rule of thumb for every diet: Don't set yourself up for failure by setting your goals so high that you cannot possibly reach them. If you're a big-framed woman with heavy bones, don't expect your diet to turn you into a Victoria's Secret runway model. The truth is that you have to live in your own body. But the joy of that hard fact is that your body can be more beautiful, more responsive, and healthier if you stick to the plan you've chosen. You may never make the cover of *GQ* or the swimsuit edition of *Sports Illustrated*, but it's well within your reach to turn heads when you walk into a room or go to a clothing store and have everything you try on actually fit. The triumph comes when you reject buying a certain piece of clothing because you don't like the color, and not because it doesn't have enough pleats.

Tips to Use

Want a one-minute glimpse at how much fat your body is packing? Here are two home-grown methods for doing just that. Grab a fold of skin at your waist; if it's more than 1 inch thick, the excess is fat. Also, stand naked in front of a mirror. Jump up and watch what jiggles. Anything that jiggles that is not supposed to jiggle is fat.

What's That Mean?

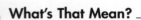

Glycogen is the stored form of glucose in the liver and muscles. It's produced when blood sugar levels are high.

You've probably read all the success stories packed into your diet book. You've been cautioned that, just because some people have lost 10 or more pounds in the first two weeks of their diet, you shouldn't expect the same result. But you can't help but hope, can you?

The first few weeks of a diet are usually a time of rapid weight loss, but each person loses differently, and many times it can be traced to a simple loss of fluid. This is cause for celebration, certainly, but save the good champagne for later. Most of this dramatic, first weight loss is because the pounds consist mainly of water and *glycogen*. Other people may not have as much fluid retained in their bodies and may not have this dramatic of an initial loss.

Over the weeks, this loss will level out. Your weight loss should stabilize at 1 to 2 pounds per week. It may not sound like much, especially if you have double—or even triple—digits to lose, but just keep reminding yourself that six months from the day you started your diet, you may be more than 20 pounds lighter.

What Should I Really Weigh?

How much should you weigh? You've already seen what the BMI chart says about your weight, and maybe that's the goal you've set yourself. People who have heavier or lighter frames, or people who are otherwise out of the norm may need a little more information.

The chart that follows details how to find out what your body frame really is. Having heavy, thick bones means you will always weigh more than someone else with lighter bones and a more delicate frame.

Get out your flexible tape measure and see where you fit in. Measure the circumference of your wrist in inches. Pick out in the table where you fall according to height, and then circle the wrist measurement that applies. Check off whether you are small-, medium-, or large-framed in one of the check boxes at the top and use it for reference.

Determining My Body Frame

My body frame is ❑ Small ❑ Medium ❑ Large

Height	Wrist Measurement
	Women
Under 5'2"	
	Small = less than 5.5"
	Medium = 5.5" to 5.7"
	Large = over 5.7"
5'2" to 5'5"	
	Small = less than 6"
	Medium = 6" to 6.25"
	Large = over 6.25"
Over 5'5"	
	Small = less than 6.25"
	Medium = 6.25" to 6.5"
	Large = over 6.5"
	Men
Over 5'5"	
	Small = 5.5" to 6.5"
	Medium = 6.5" to 7.5"
	Large = over 7.5"

All these tools will help point you in the right direction of what your goal weight or "natural" weight should be. This is the weight at which your body feels best, is healthiest, and tends to stay at. This may not be the weight you carried throughout high school and always dreamed of getting back to. The problem with that nostalgic desire is that you're older, your body is different—and probably slower, hormonally more erratic, and less resilient—than that high-rev machine you were years ago. Your body may "want" to stay at a higher weight, and that's the compromise you have to make.

One of the most life-changing activities you will do as part of your diet is start to exercise regularly. Nearly all diet plans strongly encourage a certain amount of exercise. Why? Revving up your metabolism by exercising regularly helps you lose weight and avoid the stalls and plateaus that can frustrate dieters.

Exercise also helps in the most basic of ways—it makes your body look better, sleeker, and firmer. It helps your heart and it helps your outlook, but we'll discuss exercising in much greater detail in Chapter 4.

Beware of the Initial Glitches

You may have been heavy for a long time—years, and even decades. You're used to looking in the mirror and seeing your same old heavy body looking back at you. When you start your diet, you might think the pounds will fall off in a balanced, measured way from each part of your body at the same time. That's not always the case.

Individuality is the pin that punctures that balloon. Each person responds to his or her diet in a unique way. Many people will see the weight loss first when they notice their faces—and not much else—becoming thinner.

Others will see their weight loss creep down their bodies—first the head, and then the chest will become thinner, and then the waist, then the hips, and, finally, the legs.

Tips to Use

Many diets want you to weigh yourself. The frequency varies a great deal, but the thing to remember is that not everything you see on the bathroom scale reflects the amount of fat on your body.

When you begin exercising, you might notice a jump in the scale even though you're sticking tightly to your diet. You may get frustrated that you're not losing any weight. That's the time to ask yourself these questions: Do my clothes fit looser? Am I stronger? Am I leaner? If the answer to these questions is yes, then you're likely losing fat while gaining muscle, a desirable tradeoff even though muscle, volume for volume, is heavier. In short, don't be discouraged. You might also consider weighing yourself at longer intervals than you normally would.

Now that you've mined virtually every piece of information from your past, you're ready to take a step into your present.

Take a few days—even a week—to look at what you're eating right now. Sure, you're eager to change your whole life, but take the time to set your baseline. Your motivation right now is extremely high. You're going to lose, and you're going to stick to your plan. But in the coming months, there will be those days when you feel that just one plate of french fries can't be all that bad, and what could be so wrong about that dish of chocolate fudge ice cream with just a little bit of sprinkles on top?

When you're going weak in the knees, thinking about the yummy food that got you where you are, just turn back to this page, and you will catch a glimpse of the Old You. And this Old You is the person you don't want to see ever again staring at you in the bathroom mirror.

The following pre-diet food diary will be the last gasp of your old dietary ways. In the future you can turn back to this diary to take your dietary temperature—to see whether you're falling into your old ways or how far you are going in your new lifestyle change. Seeing where you've been will help you get where you want to be.

Fill in everything you eat, and then find the nutrient values that apply to your diet in the nutrition table in Appendix C. Note the following:

> C = Calorie
>
> P = Protein
>
> DC = Digestible carbohydrate (total carbohydrate minus dietary fiber)
>
> F = Fat

Substitute PT (Points), EX (Exchanges), or whatever other measurement your diet requires for one of the categories you aren't tracking. Check off each box under Water as you drink each 8-ounce glass. Check the Vitamin box if you've taken your vitamin today.

Pre-Diet: What I'm Eating

Monday

Water
☐ ☐ ☐ ☐ ☐ ☐ ☐

Vitamin
Yes ☐

	C	P	DC	F
Breakfast				
_____	___	___	___	___
_____	___	___	___	___
Lunch				
_____	___	___	___	___
_____	___	___	___	___
Dinner				
_____	___	___	___	___
_____	___	___	___	___
Snacks				
_____	___	___	___	___
_____	___	___	___	___
TOTALS	___	___	___	___

Tuesday

Water
☐ ☐ ☐ ☐ ☐ ☐ ☐

Vitamin
Yes ☐

	C	P	DC	F
Breakfast				
_____	___	___	___	___
_____	___	___	___	___
Lunch				
_____	___	___	___	___
_____	___	___	___	___
Dinner				
_____	___	___	___	___
_____	___	___	___	___
Snacks				
_____	___	___	___	___
_____	___	___	___	___
TOTALS	___	___	___	___

Wednesday

Water   Vitamin

❑ ❑ ❑ ❑ ❑ ❑ ❑   Yes ❑   C   P   DC   F

Breakfast

	C	P	DC	F
_____	—	—	—	—
_____	—	—	—	—

Lunch

	C	P	DC	F
_____	—	—	—	—
_____	—	—	—	—

Dinner

	C	P	DC	F
_____	—	—	—	—
_____	—	—	—	—

Snacks

	C	P	DC	F
_____	—	—	—	—
_____	—	—	—	—

TOTALS   —   —   —   —

Thursday

Water   Vitamin

❑ ❑ ❑ ❑ ❑ ❑ ❑   Yes ❑   C   P   DC   F

Breakfast

	C	P	DC	F
_____	—	—	—	—
_____	—	—	—	—

Lunch

	C	P	DC	F
_____	—	—	—	—
_____	—	—	—	—

Dinner

	C	P	DC	F
_____	—	—	—	—
_____	—	—	—	—

Snacks

	C	P	DC	F
_____	—	—	—	—
_____	—	—	—	—

TOTALS   —   —   —   —

Friday

Water   Vitamin

☐ ☐ ☐ ☐ ☐ ☐ ☐   Yes ☐   C   P   DC   F

Breakfast

	C	P	DC	F
_____	—	—	—	—
_____	—	—	—	—

Lunch

	C	P	DC	F
_____	—	—	—	—
_____	—	—	—	—

Dinner

	C	P	DC	F
_____	—	—	—	—
_____	—	—	—	—

Snacks

	C	P	DC	F
_____	—	—	—	—
_____	—	—	—	—
TOTALS	—	—	—	—

Saturday

Water   Vitamin

☐ ☐ ☐ ☐ ☐ ☐ ☐   Yes ☐   C   P   DC   F

Breakfast

	C	P	DC	F
_____	—	—	—	—
_____	—	—	—	—

Lunch

	C	P	DC	F
_____	—	—	—	—
_____	—	—	—	—

Dinner

	C	P	DC	F
_____	—	—	—	—
_____	—	—	—	—

Snacks

	C	P	DC	F
_____	—	—	—	—
_____	—	—	—	—
TOTALS	—	—	—	—

Sunday

Water   Vitamin
☐ ☐ ☐ ☐ ☐ ☐ ☐   Yes ☐   C   P   DC   F

Breakfast

	C	P	DC	F
———	——	——	——	——
———	——	——	——	——

Lunch

	C	P	DC	F
———	——	——	——	——
———	——	——	——	——

Dinner

	C	P	DC	F
———	——	——	——	——
———	——	——	——	——

Snacks

	C	P	DC	F
———	——	——	——	——
———	——	——	——	——

TOTALS

The Least You Need to Know

◆ Take your medical history; knowing your medications, your family ailments, and other background information will guide you in your diet and when you talk to your doctor.

◆ Your body measurements will set a baseline, so you can better see how you're doing on your diet.

◆ Check with your doctor before starting your diet to see if you need any specialized tests or if you have to modify the diet.

◆ Record all your test results and doctor and insurance contact information, so you or a relative will have it handy in an emergency.

◆ Keep a one-week food diary before you start on your diet to help you see where you are now and, later, how far you have come.

2

Ready ... Set ... Lose!

In This Chapter

- ◆ Expecting the unexpected when starting a diet
- ◆ Understanding your body's reactions
- ◆ Beating the diet blues
- ◆ Short-circuiting a binge
- ◆ Planning meals and buying foods
- ◆ Decoding food labels

You've thrown out all the chocolate, scattered the potato chips to the four winds, and dumped all the margarine. Any foods that your diet cautions you to avoid are now either sitting on your spouse's plate, buried deep in the garbage can, or are inside the dog.

You've cleared the decks, and now you might be wondering what the coming few weeks will hold for you. You've read all the promises and glowing stories from your diet book, but you're also aware that there are times when even the best-intended of experts may put in a few too many exclamation points.

In this chapter, you'll learn how your body will likely react to a change in eating habits. You'll also learn the skills you need to carry through on your diet: from how to plan your meals and shop for food to how to detect if food labels are hiding secrets. And if you think you don't need any guidance in the grocery store after years of strolling the aisles, the FDA has some tips and suggestions that might be a surprise for you. You'll learn how to read a food nutrition label and realize that free, low, reduced, and other claims on the label may not mean what you think they mean.

> **Check This Out**
>
> Know how to tell when an apple is really fresh? Put it in water. A fresh apple will float because one-quarter of its volume is air.

This chapter also outlines how to choose the best meat, seafood, and fruits and vegetables, and gives tips on what to watch out for before you buy.

You'll see how to size up what a real serving should look like, and you'll have handy forms for recording your favorite recipes and food lists. They are convenient to take with you when you go to the store.

Many diets present you with a mouthful-by-mouthful menu plan for the first week or so. Other diets are more flexible. However rigorous or relaxed your program is, though, most diets have many things in common. This chapter will be your personal guidebook through your first few weeks.

> **Check This Out**
>
> Three main reasons for Americans becoming obese are because they eat out more, are eating larger portions, and are eating more salty snacks, soft drinks, and pizza, according to a February 2004 report from the Centers for Disease Control and Prevention (CDC). In fact, since 1971, the average daily calorie intake increased by more than 150 calories for women and more than 330 calories for men.

Off to a Fast Start

One diet doctor tells the story of one of his followers who lost 30 pounds in 60 days. A different doctor relates how a 335-pound man lost 21 pounds in the first two weeks of a diet, and how a 280-pound man lost nearly 4 pounds a week for almost three months.

It's impossible not to be buoyed by these stories and to see yourself stepping on your own scale and having your jaw drop at the plummeting numbers. It's a nice thought, it's an ideal dream, but that kind of weight loss is not the norm.

Don't set yourself up for failure by telling yourself that you're going to lose that much just as rapidly as the people in the diet book stories did. The reason the anecdotes are in the diet books in the first place is because their stories are dramatic and not typical. The truth is that nearly every single expert explains that you will lose an average of 1 to 2 pounds a week over time, a rate that is acknowledged by nutritionists to be an ideal loss.

So why do some people have dramatic initial stories? Some diets, such as low-carb plans, are naturally *diuretic,* flushing much of the retained water from your system and accounting for some of the dip in the bathroom scale. Other loss during this time may come because the levels in your body of stored sugar (*glycogen*) may be lowering.

What's That Mean?

Diuretic is a substance that tends to increase the amount of urine passed by the body.

Glycogen is made from glucose (one of the simplest forms of sugar) in the liver and muscles when blood sugar levels are high.

Who Put the Brakes On?

Even if you're one of the lucky ones who lost easily in the first few weeks, old hands at dieting warn newcomers that there are speed bumps ahead.

This is when, no matter how much you stick to your plan, you just can't seem to lose any weight.

This is your first stall, a period where your body is pausing after the first rush of lost weight. Some veteran dieters theorize that this break time is the body's way of adjusting to a rapid weight loss.

The trick, if you have this fits-and-starts style of losing weight, is to look back on the entire time you've been dieting and figure out how much weight you've lost per week, on average. If you lost 10 pounds in the first two weeks and then stall and lose nothing for the next three weeks, you will still have lost an average of 2 pounds per week, which is a desirable rate.

Blood Pressure Might Drop

Although experts don't claim that your blood pressure will drop—especially to levels where you won't need your medication—researchers strongly feel there is a link between being overweight and having high blood pressure (*hypertension*).

What's That Mean?

Hypertension is when your blood goes through your vessels with a force greater than normal. The pressure from this force can strain your heart and injure your arteries.

This is another good reason to keep track of your vital statistics on the forms in this book. If you're one of the lucky ones whose weight loss means lower blood pressure, you'll want to know it—and possibly tell your doctor who might want to adjust your medicine.

Check This Out

Seasoned low-carb dieters say that toward the end of the first month of dieting, you're probably going to hit a stall and temporarily stop losing weight.

Also, low-carb diet authors strongly feel that there is a definite link between constantly high insulin levels in the blood and high blood pressure. The focus of all low-carb diets is to lower blood insulin. If you lower blood insulin levels by not eating foods that turn into sugar, cells are not being hit with the constant demand to rid the blood of sugar. Basically, the body's blood chemistry calms down.

The Incredible Shrinking Body

Remember all those body measurements you took? They'll come in handy in the coming weeks. Although these measurements probably won't change much day to day, you'll start noticing a difference when you fill in the once-a-month diet journal form that includes your picture.

Like many dieters, you might see some body parts shrink and others stay the same because you're losing weight unevenly. Don't worry about this; it will all level out in the long run. That said, you should keep your expectations under control. For example, if you and everyone else in your family have heavy thighs, chances are that this will not only be the last place you'll lose, but those thighs may always look larger than you want them to. That's just a personal reality you'll have to live with. However, if you're looking at your family portrait right now and are thinking about all those jowls, chubby cheeks, and thick waists that are staring back at you, stop looking at the drawbacks. What you should be thinking about is how great you're going to look in your *next* family portrait.

Your diet is not about the perfect body; it's about a healthy, fit body that you can be proud of.

Check This Out

Some low-carb dieters might feel more tired, slightly euphoric, or even light-headed just after they start their diet. Why? One reason could be that the diet is working too well. Their metabolism may not be keeping pace with their weight loss. In other words, they're losing weight so fast that minerals and water may be getting depleted. The solution: Slow down the weight loss by adding a few carbs until your body adjusts.

Just for Women

Don't be surprised if right after you start your diet, your period changes. Although science is largely silent on the subject, some women who have opted for certain types of diets say that their diet disrupts their cycles in the short term. If you are one of these women, your cycle may become erratic, it may last longer or become shorter, or may become heavier or lighter. After a few months, however, your period should become normal again. This doesn't happen to every woman, but it is sometimes a side effect of dieting. If your cycle doesn't return to normal after a few months, you should talk to your doctor; it might be a sign of some other condition.

Women should also be aware that changes in their cycle may mean changes in both their measurements and their weight that have nothing to do with gaining or losing fat. Water retention at certain times of the month is just a fact of life, but one that passes fairly quickly, so if you're disappointed one day, just remember that the sudden weight gain may have nothing to do with your diet.

Check This Out

Women, prepare yourself for a parallel cycle of weight loss: two weeks where losing may be relatively easy, followed by two weeks where losing is difficult. The easy two weeks usually start on the first day of your period, and the second two weeks start after ovulation. Many women report being hungrier and having more cravings during the second two weeks. This pattern doesn't happen to every woman, but it happens often enough that you should be aware of it.

Be Gone Migraines and Headaches!

Many people say that their migraines or recurring headaches get better after they start their diet. Others say they actually began to *get* headaches.

There may be several things at play. For people who say their headaches disappeared, it might be that cutting down on processed foods, caffeine, sugar, and additives—the basic advice of nearly every diet plan—eliminated the triggers that caused the headaches.

Diet Alert

Common headache triggers: smoked or cured cheese, red wine, chocolate, fermented foods such as yogurt, nitrites or nitrate-containing foods such as cold cuts, and copper-rich foods such as nuts and shellfish.

However, if you suddenly develop headaches, take a hard look at your food journals and see what you've been eating. One person who started to get migraines on his diet suddenly realized he was eating a lot of foods with *nitrites* (such as *MSG*, the flavor enhancer common in Chinese food) and other additives. What were these foods? Deli-style cold cuts, ham, bacon, and sausage. When he eliminated these foods, the migraines went away.

What's That Mean?

Nitrites are chemicals used to enhance color and flavor and are also used as preservatives, mainly to prevent botulism. All cured meats, such as bacon, contain nitrites.

MSG is short for monosodium glutamate and is used as a flavor enhancer. MSG is made in a fermenting process that uses starch, sugar beets, sugar cane, or molasses. In the last three decades, people have reported such reactions to it as worsened asthma and headaches.

It never hurts to be tested for food intolerances, as well. If you develop headaches on your diet, and you can't figure out what's causing them, ask your doctor to test for specific allergies. You may be surprised to find out that the foods you've loved your entire life have not loved you back.

When the Scale Just Won't Budge

Truly the most dreaded time of your diet is the almost inevitable stage at which absolutely nothing seems to be happening. No matter how well you seem to be following the diet, no weight is coming off.

Timing is everything. Various experts and dieters have different views about the plateaus and stalls of "nothing happening." Generally, though, you're on a plateau when your weight, your body measurements, and your body fat have not changed for a month or more. Any less time is a stall.

Many people find that it helps to see where they are in their diets in a visual way. We've provided a weight-time graph form called Graphing My Weight Loss in Appendix B. This page is where you can chart daily, weekly, or however often you choose, a profile of how your weight loss is going.

It's like the old graphs you used to plot when you were in high school geometry. The dots are where your weight is at a certain point in time. Connect the dots over time, and you'll be able to see graphically if you're in a stall or plateau.

Note that many dieters say looking at a graph, a visual picture of their diet, derails discouragement and keeps them on their diets even when they seem to be in a horizonless plateau.

Check This Out

Some diet authors think calories are important, others do not. Either way, it never hurts to know exactly what you're eating.

- 1 gram of fat = 9 calories
- 1 gram of carbohydrate = 4 calories
- 1 gram of protein = 4 calories

Why Am I Not Losing Weight?

This is the million-dollar question. Unfortunately, there is no pat answer. Every person will have his or her own stumbling blocks, including health and medication issues or drifting off of the diet, many times without even realizing it.

If you've stalled, do not get so frustrated that you find comfort in a local restaurant's all-you-can-eat buffet table. Some calmness and clear-headed thinking when you first hit a wall will get you moving faster than you might think.

What constitutes the calm approach? First of all, take inventory:

♦ Have you started any new medications (this includes hormone therapy and birth control pills)?

♦ Has your lifestyle changed recently so that your exercise and eating routines have been disrupted? (More stress on the job? At home? Major deadlines?)

♦ Have you added a food that might be triggering a reaction? (Look in your food journals for new foods that coincide with your stall.)

♦ Have you gone off of your plan, even if you think you only "cheated" a little bit?

If the answer to any of these questions is yes, then you may be looking at the root of your stall.

Also consider food intolerances. They can cause any number of symptoms, including skin breakouts, breathing problems, joint pain, and other reactions. Common foods that can cause these problems are anything made with wheat, and such dairy products as milk, eggs, and cheese. Some diet experts think that eating foods that cause a minor allergic reaction upsets the insulin and blood sugar levels and can lead to intense cravings. Intense cravings often lead to overeating, and that may be what's causing your stall.

If you think a food is triggering any kind of reaction, go over your daily journals carefully and see if you can pinpoint the cause. Keeping your journal faithfully is the cornerstone of successful dieting.

The Salt Connection

The body is a thrifty creature. In prehistoric days when food was unpredictable, high levels of insulin meant there was plenty of food around, and this pancreatic hormone would signal the body to retain sodium so that the body would retain moisture, make more cholesterol, and store fat. The body thinks it's doing you a favor by saving up all these nutrients for the lean times ahead. Unfortunately, there's no way to tell your body that, in these modern times of gigantic portions and spectacular waste, there's no need to be so thrifty.

Because food labels seem to tell you all about milligrams and not common measurements, how do you translate that to teaspoons? Here's the key (numbers in milligrams have been rounded):

- ¼ teaspoon salt = 580 mg sodium
- ½ teaspoon salt = 1,160 mg sodium
- ¾ teaspoon salt = 1,740 mg sodium
- 1 teaspoon salt = 2,325 mg sodium

> **Check This Out**
>
> Picture what a level teaspoon of salt looks like. Now picture it sprinkled over a bunch of freshly steamed asparagus. If that's the amount of salt you're consuming every day, you're getting too much sodium, and you're putting yourself at risk for diseases such as high blood pressure.

The Institute of Medicine of the National Academies suggests that healthy adults need to consume at least 1,500 mg of sodium but not more than 2,300 mg each day.

Here's a word to the wise: Look at food labels. If you see any ingredient with some form of the word "sodium" in it, you can bet that that's exactly what's in it. For example, look for terms such as "sodium nitrate" or "monosodium glutamate." They contain sodium.

Some foods may surprise you with the amount of salt they contain. In fact, salt isn't even No. 1 in sodium on the list of the U.S. Department of Agriculture's National Nutrient Database for Standard Reference. The food with the most salt per portion in it is one packet of dried onion soup mix. It has 3,493 mg of sodium. The following table gives you an idea of other foods whose sodium content might come as something of a shock.

> **Check This Out**
>
> One of the first reactions your body will have if you're on a low-carb diet is to release water. What can happen after a few months is that your body adjusts for the low levels of sodium and becomes more responsive to it. This means that if you eat something salty, it might turn up as an unexpected weight gain, even by the next day.

The Salt Surprise

Food	Portion Size	Sodium*
Bread crumbs, seasoned	1 cup	3,180
Sauerkraut, canned (incl. liquid)	1 cup	1,560
Shrimp; breaded, fried	6–8 shrimp	1,446

continues

The Salt Surprise (continued)

Food	Portion Size	Sodium*
Potato salad; homemade	1 cup	1,322
Canned tomato sauce	1 cup	1,283
Canned stewed tomatoes	1 cup	563
Roasted ham; lean, cured	3 oz.	1,127
Low-fat cottage cheese	1 cup	917
Regular cottage cheese	1 cup	850
Soy sauce	1 TB.	914
Teriyaki sauce	1 TB.	690
Dill pickles	1 pickle	833
Tuna salad	1 cup	824
Canned Atlantic sardines	3 oz.	429
Roast turkey	3 oz.	578
Beef hot dog	1 hot dog	513
Blue cheese	1 oz.	395
Swiss cheese	1 oz.	388
Feta cheese	3 oz.	316
Cheddar cheese	1 oz.	176
Salami	2 slices	372
Chocolate milkshake	10.6 fl. oz.	333
Pork sausage	2 links	195

All sodium counts are in milligrams

Tricks to Get Yourself Unstuck

If you've gone over all your journals and figured out that neither going off the program nor gaining muscle weight is to blame for your stall, there are still some things to try before tearing out your hair and yelling at the scale.

The first thing to try: Cut back on the overall quantity of food you're eating.

You may not be drinking enough water. Oddly enough, drinking water helps you flush your kidneys and lose some water weight. This may be enough to get you started losing again. Or, if you're on a low-carb diet, you may have mistakenly picked up low-fat foods at the supermarket. Most of the time, these foods make up for the missing flavor of fat by adding fillers and carbohydrates.

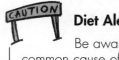

Diet Alert

Be aware that the most common cause of stalling is simply not following your diet.

Try cutting back on artificial sweeteners such as aspartame. Although no one knows why, some people seem to have a hard time losing weight if they're eating or drinking too much of these substances. Condiments, too, can be a trap. One tablespoon of ketchup, for example, has more than 26 grams of carbohydrates and 16 calories, and one tablespoon of sweet pickle relish has nearly 5 grams of carbohydrates and 20 calories.

Coffee, tea, and other caffeine-laden foods and drinks might cause a dip in your blood sugar, sparking cravings that may make you overeat. Not stopping at the coffee shop on the way to work might be hard, but it also may help get your weight loss started again.

Don't forget the web. Support groups are an invaluable resource. Be aware, though, that for the most part, people on these Internet bulletin boards and chat rooms are not doctors; they can tell you their experiences, but their own personal stories should never be taken as sound medical advice. Every diet expert urges you to remember that people's bodies react differently even if they are on the same diet. On the other hand, if you see a suggestion that looks promising, investigate it, but look before you leap.

If all else fails, you can try going back to Square One. This means going back to the first, most rigorous phase of your diet. Many people find that this is the nudge they need to move off the plateau.

Diet Alert

Before you take advice from anyone off the Internet, ask your doctor about the suggestion.

Tips to Beat the Diet Blues

Plateaus, stalls, going back to the beginning, not seeing progress, eating the same foods all the time, watching religiously what you eat—at a certain point all the care your diet demands may be a bit too demanding. You're tired of all the attention losing weight takes. You may even be bored.

How do you keep diet fatigue at bay?

- **Start cooking.** You don't have to be a graduate of *Le Cordon Bleu* to try a new recipe.

- **Enlist your family.** Make a list of everything they can do to help you, including giving you compliments and keeping you company while you exercise. In addition to helping your diet, you may get to know your family on an entirely new level.

- **Look back at the first picture you took of yourself before you started the diet**. The difference you see between then and now should be enough incentive to continue.

- **Remember your goals and dreams.** Putting yourself in the same frame of mind as when you started can elevate your desire to keep on with it.

- **Re-read your diet book.** It may have been awhile since you looked through the success stories, the encouraging remarks, and the tips that each diet plan offers. Revisit these and find your old enthusiasm.

- **Sample other diets.** Many dieters have found that, as they go along, they become less of a purist about one single diet plan. If something from another diet intrigues you, try it. There are no Diet Police who will come for you if you borrow from other plans, and the mix may be just what you need to stay interested.

- **Shake up your eating habits.** Change the time of day you eat each meal, or eat frequent mini-meals instead of the larger, less-often ones.

- **Try a new exercise.** If your exercise routine is, well, routine, try doing something else. If you always walk to the mini-mart and back before dinner, try bicycling to a different destination.

- **Go dancing.** With country-western line dancing still popular, you don't even need a partner. There's nothing more refreshing than vigorous exercise that feels like fun, not work.

- **Reward yourself for good behavior.** Give yourself a gift when you reach personal milestones.

We've even provided a few gift certificates for you. All you have to do is fill in your name, the date, and the reward you're giving yourself.

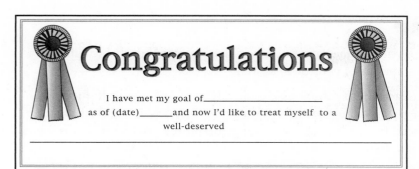

Reward yourself.

Reached a milestone? Overcame an obstacle? Broke through a plateau? Or maybe you just feel proud of yourself for sticking with your diet. Reward yourself. Fill out this gift certificate, and treat yourself right. You deserve to be recognized. It's a good idea to make a few copies of this page; you'll need more certificates as you pass even more milestones.

Binges

The darker side of plateaus and stalls is the binge. If you've ever risen out of bed at midnight, walked like one possessed to the refrigerator, and eaten everything from the shelves that couldn't escape from you, you know what these defeating episodes are.

Your best bet is to be prepared to deal with the urges before they happen.

What Triggers a Binge?

The best plan is, of course, to head the binge off before it starts. How to do that?

- ◆ **Make sure you take your vitamins regularly.** If you are hit by an irresistible craving, it just may be your body's way of telling you it needs a certain nutrient.

- ◆ **Drink plenty of water.** Your body can get confused and mistake thirst for hunger.

- ◆ **Get some sleep.** Everybody's need is different, and if you're bright-eyed on six hours, that's fine. When you're tired, your ability to resist temptation is usually the first thing that flies out the window.

- ◆ **Avoid what causes a binge.** This could be anything from office birthday parties to that one piece of delectable chocolate you swore you'd never have again. It's the slippery slope you don't even want to put a foot on.

Tips to Brake the Binge

The following list provides some suggestions we like, and you'll probably come up with some creative solutions of your own, as well.

◆ **Control the chaos.** If you absolutely, positively can't help yourself, then pick your binge. Slap your hands away from the chocolate, cookies, and ice cream and reach instead for protein and fat. A binge on protein and fat will satisfy you a lot longer than desserts and sweets.

◆ **Pinpoint your trigger foods.** If the smell of potato chips induces a trance of pigging out, then this is a trigger food. Figure out the foods you really can't resist and cut them out altogether, or plan on a portion of them as a once-in-a-while treat.

◆ **Calm down.** Stress is a common trigger. Take a yoga class and learn those ancient relaxation techniques. Or make a deal with yourself to binge but only after you go for a walk or a bike ride. After you've exercised, many times the urge to binge has faded.

> **Check This Out**
>
> Eat nuts. Unless you're allergic to them or react in some other way, a good bet to head off a binge is eating such foods as macadamias, walnuts, Brazil nuts, and pecans. They're high in fat, satisfying, and help control blood sugar levels. And they're one snack you can carry with you that won't leak, melt, or get everything gooey. One caution: Nuts tend to be low in carbohydrates but high in calories, so adjust according to what type of diet you are on.

◆ **Fool your craving.** If you can't stop drooling in the ice cream aisle at the supermarket, and you know disaster is just a checkout line away, opt for the diet-friendly version of the food. It will probably satisfy your craving and not take you too far off of your plan.

◆ **Drink water.** We know, we know, we've said this so many times before, but the reason we keep saying it is because it really works.

◆ **Let yourself off the hook.** A binge just means you put more food in your mouth than you should have. No one has died; nothing has happened that you can't fix. Of all the crimes you could commit, bingeing is the most forgivable. And the best way to forgive yourself is to get right back on your diet.

The Nuts and Bolts of Your First Week

If you're used to throwing something in the microwave, noshing all day on anything that comes in a glossy bag, and having the raging munchies at 11 P.M., well, all that spontaneity is great, but it's also probably what packed on all those extra pounds you want to lose. So, your new diet is about changing habits, and one of those habits you're leaving behind is disorganized eating. Your diet is about regular meals and snacks that are figured out in advance. Or, if they're not precisely figured out, your meals are at least prepared with "legal" foods in your cupboards and a few fallback plans in the form of already-made dishes in your refrigerator and freezer.

This well-stocked kitchen begins with the basics: meat, seafood, fruits and vegetables, and oils. And you have to know what you're buying, or you may sabotage your plan at its very foundation.

Picking Your Meat

Diet experts urge their followers to opt for lean cuts of beef, lamb, pork, and other meats, and even suggest choosing wild game or free-range-type meats that are naturally less fatty and free of antibiotics and other chemical enhancements.

There are three main grades of beef: Prime, Choice, and Select. Prime is the most tender and juiciest, but it also has the most fat. Your best bet is to skip this grade of meat and choose from the two lower ones. Choice meat is high quality but has less fat (marbling). Roasts and steaks from the most tender parts, the loin and rib, are good for dry-roasting. Rump, round, and blade chuck are less tender cuts but can also be dry-roasted.

Check This Out

Fat still matters even on a low-carb diet, and you have to keep it in proportion with the carbohydrates and proteins you are eating. Ground beef comes in a variety of fat content. A patty of cooked, extra-lean hamburger has 14 grams of total fat, compared with a regular patty that has 17 grams.

If you're really trying to watch the fat in your diet, and you can't decide whether to eat that hamburger you just bought or throw it away for something leaner, try this. Sauté the hamburger and then rinse it under warm running water for 30 seconds. This last-minute shower will remove the extra fat.

Select meat is the leanest of the three retail grades of beef and usually lacks the tenderness and juiciness of the higher grades. You're better off marinating these cuts before cooking or cooking them with moisture to get the most flavor and tenderness from them.

> **Check This Out**
>
> Pork chops, with or without bones, come from cuts such as center loin, rib chops, or sirloin chops, and are tasty prepared almost any way. Rib cuts, such as spareribs and back ribs, are best when slow-cooked. Spareribs come from the belly of the animal, while back ribs come from the loin.

Pork meat tends to be so uniformly leaner than it was decades ago, that the USDA only grades it Acceptable and Unacceptable. Most of the visible fat is trimmed off at the processing plant, and the animals are also bred to be leaner. Look for cuts that have a small amount of fat on the outside, a little marbling, is firm to the touch, and grayish-pink in color. Tenderloins are the juiciest and most tender of the cuts and are extremely lean.

Lamb comes from animals less than a year old, and the best cuts are graded Prime and Choice. Mutton comes from sheep that are older than a year and does not have a Prime grade.

The same general principles apply here that did to beef. Prime is the juiciest and the most flavorful, but also contains the most fat. Choice has less marbling than Prime but is still high quality. The less tender cuts are the breast, riblets, neck, and shank, and these cuts are good for stews, curries, or other such lamb dishes.

Storing the meat after you get it home is also important. Meat frozen at 0°F can be kept for a long time—up to 12 months for some beef cuts and up to 2 months for pork sausage. Fresh meat will only keep a matter of days in the refrigerator, which should be no warmer than 40°F. Fresh pork sausage will only keep 1 to 2 days in the refrigerator, while fresh beef steaks will keep from 3 to 5 days.

When cooking, be aware that illness-causing pathogens, including Escherichia coli O157:H7, will die when heated to a temperature of 160°F. And don't be fooled by the color of, say, ground beef. Studies have shown that even if your cooked hamburger looks brown, it may only be heated to internal temperatures as low as 131°F. Use a temperature thermometer to be sure your meat is heated high enough to kill harmful bacteria.

Safe Cooking Temperatures (in Degrees Fahrenheit)

Pork	Ground Beef	Whole Poultry and Thighs	Ground Poultry Breasts	Chicken or Turkey
160	160	180	170	165

The Best Fish and Shellfish

Nearly every diet touts the health benefits of seafood, particularly fish that are rich in the polyunsaturated fat omega-3. This fatty acid especially helps keep your heart healthy, cuts the risk of plaques in your arteries, lowers triglyceride levels, and it can even slightly lower your blood pressure.

The best way to get more omega-3 in your diet is to eat such fatty fish as mackerel, sardines, tuna, salmon, and other such fish. If you don't have much experience preparing fresh seafood, there are a few tricks you should know.

> **Check This Out**
>
> The next time you're strolling by the fish counter at the supermarket, take a whiff. If you smell anything but salt and ice, then you may want to take your business elsewhere. Fresh fish should not smelly fishy.

Here are some tips for buying seafood:

- **Buy it last.** It's very perishable, and if you can't get it home within an hour, be sure you have a cooler you can store it in while you're traveling.

- **Buy from a retailer you trust.** Don't buy seafood from the back of a pickup truck parked by the side of the road—you won't know if the seafood has been properly handled or have any idea how long it's been in the back of that truck.

- **Look the fish in the eye.** Whole fish should have bright, clear eyes, and a clear cornea. The older the fish, the more the eyes become pink and cloudy. The gills should be bright red and have no slime. The flesh should be firm to the touch.

- **Inspect the edges of fillets.** The edges of fish fillets should not be brown or dry.

- **Tap and smell those mollusks.** The shells of live mussels, clams, or oysters should be plump and have no strong odor. You can tell if they are alive by tapping on the shells; they will close tightly. If the shell is open, the seafood is probably dead, and you shouldn't eat it.

- **Feel and smell the scallops.** Scallops are shucked at sea and not sold live. They should be firm and smell sweet.

- **Look for signs of life in crustaceans.** Live crabs, lobsters, and crayfish should still be moving even if they are refrigerated. If they're not moving, they're dead. After these shellfish are dead, bacteria start growing, and eating them may make you sick.

- ◆ **Check the color, feel, and smell of shrimp.** Raw shrimp should be firm, smell mild, and be white-colored with hints of pink and red.

- ◆ **Skip the case showing raw and cooked seafood.** Don't buy cooked seafood, such as shrimp, if it is in the same display case as raw fish. The cooked seafood might become contaminated.

- ◆ **Avoid damaged goods.** If frozen seafood packages are open, torn, or crushed, don't buy them. Don't buy frozen seafood that is kept above the frost line in the grocery store's freezer. If there is frost or ice crystals, it may mean the seafood has been stored a long time or has been frozen, thawed, and refrozen.

After you have your seafood home, put it in the coldest part of the refrigerator—in a meat compartment or right under the freezer. Don't pack it in tightly with other foods but allow air to circulate around the package. If live shellfish die or their shells break or crack while they're being stored, throw them away.

It also helps when you shop to have a visual idea of how much food one serving would be. Diets are fairly uniform when it comes to serving size, but make sure you consult your book for specifics. The following table will give you a general idea.

How Big Is a Serving?

Food	Quantity	Is Like …
Butter	1 tsp.	Postage stamp
Salad Dressing	2 TB.	Ping-pong ball
Yogurt	1 cup	Softball
Cheese	1 oz.	4 dice
Leafy veg.	1 cup	Softball
Chopped veg.	½ cup	Half an orange
Meat, fish	3 oz.	Deck of cards
Peanut butter	2 TB.	Golf ball
Fruit	1 medium	Tennis ball

Sources: U.S. Department of Health and Human Services, the National Heart, Lung, and Blood Institute, and the Colorado Department of Public Health and Environment

Not All Fruits and Vegetables Are Created Equal

Every diet will have slightly different dos and don'ts, but all encourage eating green, leafy vegetables and urge you to be careful of the amounts of starchy vegetables you eat. Fruits also have a place in all diets, but, again, you have to pick and choose the ones that fit your plan best.

Also, many diets want you to restrict the eating of such dense fruits as bananas and papayas.

After you've filled your grocery cart and brought everything home, your produce still needs some tender loving care.

> **Check This Out**
>
> Form matters. For instance, The Zone low-carb diet deplores the act of juicing. Author Barry Sears says that removing the fiber from fruit by running it through a juicer is like taking the brakes off of how fast the fruit's carbohydrate enters your bloodstream. Whole fruit's fiber slows the process down, which is what a low-carb dieter wants so that insulin levels stay more stable.

- If the produce is peeled or cut, it should go straight into the refrigerator. If it has been cut and left at room temperature for more than two hours, it should be thrown away.

- Wash your hands with soap and water before and after handling the produce.

- Just before eating the produce, wash it with cool tap water, and do not use soap. Discard bruised or damaged parts of the produce before you eat it.

Here are some tips on choosing and keeping fresh fruits:

- **Apples.** The longer on the tree, the higher the sugar content. Look for firmness, fragrance, and uniformly bright color. Apples keep ripening even after they're picked. Put them in the refrigerator in a plastic bag with plenty of holes for ventilation. Store in a single layer, not piled up.

> **Check This Out**
>
> Considering the fact that an average apple has about 17.3 digestible carbs, a tree-ripened one might be an even heavier hit for those counting carbs.

- **Oranges.** A few "scars" on the peel don't affect quality. The fruit should be firm and heavy and smell citrus-y. If the fruit is shriveled or soft, don't buy it. Keep oranges at room temperature, and they'll be fine for about two weeks. Turn them often and check for mold.

◆ **Blueberries.** Buy plump berries with tight skins and deep coloring. They should look a bit dusty. They'll keep in the refrigerator for up to 10 days if you put them in a single layer on a paper towel in a covered pan. Don't wash until just before eating.

Here are some tips on choosing and keeping fresh vegetables:

◆ **Tomatoes.** Buy them with firm, bright skins. They should have a soft smell at the stem. Don't buy mushy or pale-colored tomatoes that are blemished or cracked. Don't refrigerate them until you cut them. To encourage them to ripen, put them in a paper bag with an apple for 24 hours. The bag should have plenty of holes.

◆ **Broccoli.** The clusters should be tight and dark green, and the stalks light green with a consistent thickness. You can keep it in the refrigerator crisper for 3 to 5 days.

◆ **Leafy greens.** Typical shelf life is 10 to 14 days. High humidity keeps them from wilting. Choose greens that are deeply colored with leaves that are crisp. Don't buy wilted or soft greens. Keep them in the refrigerator's crisper.

Fats—Separating the "Good" from the "Bad"

Saturated fats usually come from animals. Meat, cheese, seafood, and egg yolks are examples. This type of fat can raise your blood cholesterol levels more than simply eating high-cholesterol foods, and saturated fats tend to raise both the "good" (*HDL*) and "bad" (*LDL*) cholesterol levels at the same time.

What's That Mean?

Saturated fats are generally solid at room temperature and most often come from animal sources, although palm and coconut oils are also high in this fat. This type of fat is considered less healthy than other kinds of fat and is linked to higher blood cholesterol levels.

HDL is short for high-density lipoprotein and is nicknamed the "good" cholesterol because it can sweep away the sticky LDL cholesterol in the blood so that it doesn't adhere to blood vessels.

LDL stands for low-density lipoprotein and is usually called the "bad" cholesterol because it tends to stick to the walls of blood vessels.

The following table will help you see how your blood levels measure up (numbers represent milligrams per deciliter of blood).

Blood Cholesterol Levels

Total Cholesterol

Desirable	Borderline High	High
Less than 200	200–239	240 and above

LDL

Optimal	Near Optimal	Borderline High	High	Very High
Less than 100	100–129	130–159	160–189	190 and above

Source: National Heart, Lung, and Blood Institute

HDL should be more than 40; more than 60 will help lower the risk of heart disease.

Trans-fatty acids (trans fats) are made when liquid vegetable oil and hydrogen are heated so that the hydrogen is forced into the oil.

This hydrogenation process turns what would ordinarily be a liquid oil (corn oil, for instance) at room temperature into a solid that, with a few other modifications, can be turned into margarine. The more hydrogen permeating the oil, the harder the final product. This is why soft, tub margarine is easier to spread than a stick of margarine. The tub margarine is less hydrogenated. Processed foods of every sort are generally rich in this sort of fat. Trans fats also tend to be worse for your health than saturated fats because trans fats do two undesirable things at the same time: They raise the "bad" (LDL) cholesterol and lower the "good" (HDL) cholesterol.

The following table can help you avoid some surprising trans fat–rich foods. The figure in the Trans Fats column indicates percent of the total fat that is trans per 100 grams of food.

What's That Mean?

Trans-fatty acids are made when liquid oils are combined with hydrogen and heated to form solid fats such as shortening.

Ten Foods High in Trans-Fatty Acids

Food	Trans Fat
Snack crackers	38
Baked taco shells	32
French fries	34
Low-cal ranch dressing	13
Popcorn, oil popped	35
Beef bouillon cube	34
Chicken bouillon cube	18
Chocolate frosting	20
Granola bar w/choc	18
Cereal, wheat/bran flakes with raisins/nuts	15

Information courtesy of the U.S. Department of Agriculture

Polyunsaturated and *monounsaturated fats* come from plant sources such as olives, peanuts, and soybeans. These oils and fats are desirable because they are the flip side of trans fats. Poly- and monounsaturated oils and fats lower the "bad" cholesterol and can raise the "good" cholesterol levels in the blood.

What's That Mean?

Polyunsaturated fat is found in high concentrations in many vegetable oils such as corn, soybean, and sunflower; in nuts; and in high-fat fish such as tuna.

Monounsaturated fat is found in high concentrations in oils that include olive oil, canola oil, and peanut oil. It is linked to raising levels of "good" cholesterol and lowering levels of "bad" cholesterol.

What are these oils, and how do they rank against each other? The table that follows is a good at-a-glance aid for choosing the best kind of oil for your diet.

Also, remember that just because an oil is considered monounsaturated or polyunsaturated, that doesn't mean it is completely free of the other kinds of fat.

How Oils Stack Up

Oils	Saturated*	Monounsaturated*	Polyunsaturated*
Olive	2	10	1.5
Canola	1	8	4
Peanut	2.5	6	4
Soybean	2	3	8
Palm	7	5	1
Corn	2	3.5	8
Sunflower	1.5	6	5.5
Safflower	1	2	10
Coconut	12	1	0.5

Weight is in grams, rounded to nearest half-gram; portion size = 1 tablespoon = 13.6 grams
Information courtesy of the U.S. Department of Agriculture

Get Ready to Shop

Before you even set foot inside your car to go to the grocery store, there are several things you can do to help yourself resist the urge to indulge.

First, have something to eat. Even the most stoic of dieters will succumb to the free sugar cookies, samples of canned ham, and cheese tasters if they walk starving through those electric doors of the supermarket. If the edge is off your appetite, then you're good to go.

To the next step, that is.

Don't leave home without a shopping list. Especially in the first stages of your diet, this command is easy to follow. Your book will generally lay out what you can and cannot have, and most books have a week or more of menus and dozens of pages of recipes. Sit down, open your diet book, grab a pen, and start writing. Mark the foods that you want to have and write them—and all the ingredients it takes to make them—on your list.

If you've got some favorite recipes, or find some in your diet book, you'll want to keep them handy. The forms that follow will keep all your favorites in one convenient spot. You can even list all the ingredients you need to shop for next to those recipes. Never again go searching for how to make that great broiled lemon salmon dish or that curried chicken!

If you're on a low-carb diet, fill in the nutrient breakdown of the dish so you know the proportions. If you're on a diet that measures food with points, exchanges, or some other way, fill in those values and skip the blanks you don't need.

My Favorite Recipes

Name: _____

How to prepare:

_____
_____
_____
_____
_____
_____
_____
_____
_____
_____
_____
_____

Serving Size: _____

Carbs: _____

Protein: _____

Fat: _____

Points: _____

Shopping List:

_____
_____
_____
_____
_____
_____
_____

Name: _____

How to prepare:

_____
_____
_____
_____
_____
_____
_____
_____
_____
_____
_____
_____

Serving Size: _____

Carbs: _____

Protein: _____

Fat: _____

Points: _____

Shopping List:

_____
_____
_____
_____
_____
_____
_____

Name: _____

How to prepare:

_____

_____

_____

_____

_____

_____

_____

_____

_____

_____

_____

_____

Serving Size: _____

Carbs: _____

Protein: _____

Fat: _____

Points: _____

Shopping List:

_____

_____

_____

_____

_____

_____

_____

_____

Name: _____

How to prepare:

_____

_____

_____

_____

_____

_____

_____

_____

_____

_____

_____

_____

_____

Serving Size: _____

Carbs: _____

Protein: _____

Fat: _____

Points: _____

Shopping List:

_____

_____

_____

_____

_____

_____

_____

_____

Reading Food Labels

Everybody's seen a Nutrition Facts label. They're so common that it's easy to overlook them. Never forget these little helpers; they are going to make your life much easier on your diet. Plus, a careful reading of your food labels might be the key to kick-starting your diet if you stall.

Check This Out

Since 1990, the FDA has required nutrition labels for most foods on grocery store shelves. This covered the nutrition basics, but people began to demand more information. Saturated fat and dietary cholesterol made the labels in 1993. There are places where you may not see these labels, however. Labeling for raw produce, such as lettuce and carrots, and fish is voluntary.

You soon won't have to guess how much trans fat is in prepared food—it'll be right on the label with saturated fat, dietary fiber, cholesterol, and the other nutritional values. The FDA is requiring food makers to list trans fat on labels by January 2006.

So, everything's laid out, plain and simple. What could be so tough about reading a food label? Well, actually nothing. But you have to know exactly what you're looking at.

The basic Nutrition Facts label is straightforward enough. Take a look at the graphic that follows, and you'll see all the basic values that are covered.

The first thing to watch out for is the serving size. The print is tiny, so it's easy to miss. But it makes a big difference if that cereal you love so much and think is so diet-friendly turns out to have a serving size of just ¼ cup. You've been eating four times that, thinking you're home free and wondering why you just can't budge off that stall you're in.

Joined at the hip with the serving size is the value that tells you how many servings are in a container. This is again where you can be fooled. If you're wolfing down your favorite potato chips, amazed that they're so diet-friendly and equally amazed that you're not losing an ounce, take a look at how many servings are in that teeny, tiny bag. There may be two or more, and it may be throwing you way off your diet.

Calories, grams of fat, total carbohydrates, dietary fiber, and protein are the lines that are most important to dieters. Whatever plan you are on, look to the nutrition label to be your guide.

Nutrition Facts

Serving Size 1 cup (228g)
Serving Per Container 2

Amount Per Serving

Calories 250   Calories from Fat 110

% Daily Value*

Total Fat 12g	**18%**
Saturated Fat 3g	**15%**
Cholesterol 30mg	**10%**
Sodium 470mg	**20%**
Total Carbohydrate 31g	**10%**
Dietary Fiber 0g	**0%**
Sugars 5g	
Protein 5g	

Vitamin A	4%
Vitamin C	2%
Calcium	20%
Iron	4%

* Percent Daily Values are based on a 2,000 calorie diet. Your Daily Values may be higher or lower depending on your calorie needs:

	Calories:	2,000	2,500
Total Fat	Less than	65g	80g
Sat Fat	Less than	20g	25g
Cholesterol	Less than	300mg	300mg
Sodium	Less than	2,400mg	2,400mg
Total Carbohydrate		300g	375g
Dietary Fiber		25g	30g

Nutrition Facts label.

(Drawing courtesy of FDA)

Check This Out

Low-carb diets generally want you to subtract the amount of dietary fiber from the amount of total carbohydrates. What's left is the carbs that you count on your diet. Why? Fiber is a type of carbohydrate, but it is the part of it that your body can't digest. Fiber passes straight through. Because it doesn't affect your insulin level, it doesn't count toward your daily carb total.

Sodium also appears on the label. Be aware of the maximum you should eat daily and keep under that level.

How to Find Hidden Sugars

Now we get to the most interesting part of talking about the Nutrition Facts label: the things that can be disguised on it.

The first thing to know is that the ingredient list on your food's label has a pecking order: The most plentiful ingredient is the first one listed; the least plentiful is the last. This guide to quantity can help you make a smart decision.

Let's first consider sugar, an ingredient that all diets want you to cut down on. Pick up any food out of your cupboard. If you see any of the following listed, the food you're looking at is probably high in sugar.

- ◆ Dextrin
- ◆ Fruit juice concentrate
- ◆ Maltose
- ◆ Malt syrup
- ◆ Lactose
- ◆ Dextrose
- ◆ Fructose
- ◆ Turbinado sugar
- ◆ Treacle
- ◆ Carob

There are more than just these, but here is a clue to find others: Look for ingredients that end in -ose; they're usually sugars.

What's That Mean?

Sugar alcohols are often substitutes for sugar in food and often appear in sugar-free products. Common ones include maltitol, lactitol, xylitol, hydrogenated starch hydrolysates (HSH), and sorbitol.

Another substance that acts as sugar is the *sugar alcohol*. This substance's main claim to fame is that sugar alcohols don't cause cavities, which is why you'll see these alcohols in sugar-free chewing gum. However, sugar alcohols in food do not necessarily mean the food is low-carb or diet-friendly in general. Also, some annoying side effects from eating too many sugar alcohols can be bloating and diarrhea.

MSG is a common additive in Chinese restaurants, but it's also common to find it the foods in your own cupboard. Why is MSG so important to find? People have reported such reactions as breathing problems and headaches—and even more serious reactions from this chemical.

Even if you have no reaction to this chemical, it never hurts to know where it is on the food label. Look for any of the following: hydrolyzed food protein, hydrolyzed plant protein, hydrolyzed food starch, natural flavors, and vegetable protein. It can, of course, be listed under its own name, as well.

> **Check This Out**
>
> Some experts cite MSG as a concentrated form of sodium that can trigger various reactions that range from weight gain and cravings to tiredness and water retention.

How can you tell if there are hidden nutrients? Each gram of fat has 9 calories, each carbohydrate has 4, and each protein has 4. Find each nutrient in the food label and multiply the number of grams times the calories in each gram. The sum of these three multiplications should add up to the calorie count at the top of the food label. If the numbers aren't the same, you may have some hidden nutrients.

Is "Free" Really Free?

Low-fat, low-calorie, sodium free—there are numerous permutations of terms that describe food.

Whether you're counting carbs, calories, fat, or some other nutrient, what the following labels mean is important to keep in mind. All the definitions are based on one serving.

- ◆ **Calorie free:** Fewer than 5 calories
- ◆ **Low calorie:** 40 calories or fewer
- ◆ **Reduced calorie:** At least 25 percent fewer calories than the regular food
- ◆ **Fat free:** Less than ½ gram of fat
- ◆ **Low fat:** 3 grams of fat or less
- ◆ **Reduced fat:** At least 25 percent less fat than the regular food
- ◆ **Sodium free:** Fewer than 5 mg
- ◆ **Very low sodium:** Fewer than 35 mg
- ◆ **Low sodium:** Fewer than 140 mg
- ◆ **High fiber:** More than 5 grams

The Least You Need to Know

◆ Expect weight loss to slow and a period of adjustment for your body to take place as you continue on your diet.

◆ Periods of not losing weight are common and can be caused by changing medicines, eating too much salt, hormonal shifts, and other events.

◆ Planning meals, choosing the right foods, and knowing how to safely prepare them are key to keeping on your diet.

◆ Reading food labels can pinpoint trouble spots in your diet and even show you if nutrients are being hidden.

◆ Free, low, and reduced may not mean what you think they do on a label.

Chapter 3

Eating in the Real World

In This Chapter

- ◆ Sidestepping diet landmines
- ◆ Planning for restaurant and holiday eating
- ◆ Defusing diet emergencies before they happen
- ◆ Avoiding lapses triggered by stress and fatigue

Just when you thought it was safe to go into your refrigerator, another challenge emerges. The time will come when you have to venture out into the real world of restaurants, friends, special occasions, and oh-so-tempting foods. Before your diet, these events would have meant postprandial guilt, self-doubt, and empty promises never, never, never again to eat the rest of the chocolate fudge cheesecake on your date's plate; however, now things have changed.

In this chapter, you'll learn where all the diet landmines are buried in restaurants and at holiday and special occasion outings that you just can't avoid. This chapter will guide you past the dishes that will throw you off of your diet and steer you toward ones that will keep you on track.

You'll figure out how to triage your way through the menu by filling out a planning form that allows you to pick the foods and quantities you can have and still stick to your diet.

You'll also find out that other things—from tiredness and stress to sleep problems—can trigger a lapse in your eating habits. You'll go through a checklist of questions that will inventory how well you are sleeping and if there is a problem you should be talking about with your doctor.

Finally, you'll be given various suggestions that might help you avoid a hard fall off your diet.

Have a Seat, and Let's Eat

A white tablecloth restaurant can be the family-owned pub around the corner or the fancy French restaurant where the waiters wear white gloves and everyone addresses you as sir and madam. You have a lot of leeway here, and you can always ask the waiter if the chef can prepare a certain dish so that it will fit into your diet. Ask for broccoli or another vegetable instead of potato or rice, for instance. Keep in mind your diet's specific restrictions. If you're on The Zone, for instance, the rule is that each meal must not have more than 500 calories.

Also, because portion sizes have become so bloated these days, there are a few things you can do to help stick to your diet.

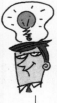

Tips to Use

Think of a buffet as an all-you-can-eat feeding trough and an invitation to diet disaster. The quantities are massive, and hidden sugars, fats, and carbohydrates are nearly everywhere. If you have no choice, you'll need every ounce of willpower to get past the dessert table and other temptations. Look for freshly carved meats, steamed vegetables, and simply prepared foods. Your best bet: Avoid buffets.

- When the waiter brings your food, immediately ask him for a take-home box. When he brings it, remove enough food so that whatever is left on your plate is the correct portion size for your diet. Close the box lid and put it out of sight. You've just removed a major amount of temptation.

- Split the meal with a companion.

- Have an idea of what you're going to order before you even walk into the restaurant.

- Skip the extras such as dinner rolls, biscuits, and crackers.

- Forego the prepared salad dressings; many times they are heavy on fat and sugar, and may tip you out of your diet. Opt, instead, for olive oil and vinegar.

- Be careful of sauces and soups; many times they are thickened with bread, potato, or flour, none of which will do your diet any good.

- Decide on your main course first; that will help you decide what you can have to fill out the rest of the meal.

- Choose simplicity. The more complex the preparation, the more likely the dish will blow your diet.

- Take a look at the Nutritive Table in Appendix C; it will tell you exactly what is in each food.

Diet Alert

Watch out for balsamic vinegar. If you're on a low-carb plan, be aware that this dark, brewed vinegar has widely varying amounts of digestible carbohydrates per tablespoon, from 0.9 grams on one brand, 3 grams on another, and even more on other brands.

Italian

For dieters, this wonderful cuisine can be frustrating. Go to an Italian restaurant and not have pasta and buttery garlic bread? Sacrilege! Well, consider this: Good Italian restaurants have other parts of the menu, as well. Let your eyes drift over to the meat, fish, salad, and appetizer sections. You don't have to have deep-fried cheese in breading (mozzarella in carozza) as an appetizer; you can have a grilled Portobello mushroom.

The best bet for any restaurant is to have a plan before you even make the reservation. Use the Game Plan form we've included for Italian cuisine to help you with other restaurants and types of food. Make plenty of copies of this blank form, so you'll have one for each place you frequent. List what you can have to drink, two or three appetizers, a salad and a dressing you can have, two or three entrees, and so on. Write down what usually comes with the entrée (a side of spaghetti in an Italian restaurant, for instance) and decide if you want to substitute a vegetable or some other diet-friendly food for it.

Check This Out

Tomato sauces can rack up quite a large score, carb-wise, because many times they have added sugar; try switching to pesto sauce instead, which has around 0.2 digestible carbohydrates per tablespoon (depending on how the basil leaves, pine nuts, garlic, parmesan, and olive oil are mixed). It's good on everything from chicken and vegetables to veal and fish.

The Game Plan

Drink: _____

Appetizer: _____

Salad & dressing: _____

Entrée: _____

_____

_____

Send back the: _____

_____

... and substitute: _____

_____

Vegetables: _____

Tips to Use _____

One of the foods to be careful of is duck. Duck dishes tend to have more fat and be topped with sweet sauces more than are other meat choices.

French

If you think French cuisine is only cream sauces and unpronounceable wines, you have a pleasant surprise in store. A French restaurant can offer some of the most diet-friendly dishes of nearly any type of cuisine. Look for—or ask the waiter for—broiled, poached, or steamed foods, including fish, which can be steamed "en papillote" (wrapped loosely in paper and baked with herbs in its own juices).

Southern

The South can pile on the carbohydrates, the calories, and the fat, and you'll hardly even be aware that those light, fluffy biscuits and creamy grits with butter are pushing you way off your diet. Also, the spiciness of such regional delights as Cajun and Creole cooking might tend to make you retain water, and the result you may quickly see on your bathroom scale.

The thing to remember here is that the South is home to some of the finest seafood cooking in the land. Ask the chef to broil or bake whenever possible, and ask for vegetable substitutes for the rice, potatoes, or grits that are served with many dishes.

Mexican

Because there is so much Mexican-style fast food around, it's easy to forget that this is a fine, often tangy cuisine that features plenty of fresh vegetables, fish, and meats that are simply prepared. The trick is to avoid the oh-so-tempting extras that appear on the table before you've even ordered. One ounce of those tortilla chips has 142 calories, 7 grams of fat, and about 16 digestible carbs—and that's before you've even dipped them in the salsa (4 calories, a trace of fat, and 0.7 digestible carbs per tablespoon).

> **Check This Out**
>
> Mexican food uses quite a bit of tomato, and, if you're watching carbohydrates, it's useful to remember that a half-cup of chopped tomato has 3 digestible carbs.

Asian

Japanese and Chinese foods tend to be generously laced with soy sauce, so you'll want to watch out for this. If you can't seem to lose any weight even though you've been eating healthy Chinese takeout, look to the soy sauce: 1 tablespoon has 871 mg of sodium, and that amount might make your body retain water.

Also, ask the waiter to skip the MSG; many people have no reaction to this flavor enhancer, but for some, it triggers cravings and other undesirable effects that can derail your diet. Oils are an integral part of these cuisines, but make sure your restaurant is cooking with the healthier peanut or sesame oils. If the oil is neither one of those, order a steamed dish instead. If you're a soup lover, you may be disappointed when you go to an Asian restaurant. Many soups are thickened with cornstarch, which can pile on the calories and carbs, so you might want to forego this course.

> **Tips to Use**
>
> One good hint for eating Asian: Try the chopsticks. You can't eat nearly as fast with them as you do with a fork and spoon. Slowing down your eating will help you eat less.

Mid-Eastern, Indian, and Greek

These cuisines have plenty of diet-friendly dishes, but there's also plenty to watch out for. Before you even get your main course, you'll probably be tempted with the flat-breads and those wonderfully puffy nan breads—stuffed or with a variety of flavorings—that appear on Indian tables. Pita or pocket breads are on the Mid-Eastern and Greek menus. Your best bet: Tell the waiter not to bring the bread at all; what's out of reach is not going into your stomach.

> **Tips to Use**
>
> Dips such as hummus (made with pureed chickpeas) and baba ghanoush (an eggplant-based dip) often accompany the table breads. You're much better off asking the waiter to take away the bread and bring you cucumbers or other vegetables you can use for the dips.

Often, in the cuisines of these regions, yogurt is used in sauces, main courses, and dressings. People on low-fat diets will welcome this ingredient in place of the more fattening cream, but low-carb dieters want to be aware that plain yogurt has 9 grams of digestible carbohydrates in ½ cup.

Fast Food Eating

When experts talk about the epidemic of obesity in this country, fingers are quick to point in the direction of fast food restaurants. As more of these restaurants came on the scene over the years, the competition for customers escalated at the same time the size of their food portions did. As hips widened, so did the outcry against doubling and tripling a normal serving size. The fast food giants are listening: By the end of 2004, McDonald's no longer routinely offered a Super Size portion at its 13,000 outlets. This means the 7-ounce Super Size fries with its 610 calories, 29 grams of fat, and 70 grams of digestible carbs has bitten the dust. However, the large fries at 540 calories, 26 grams of fat, and 62 grams of digestible carbs will still be on the menu. Other major players in the fast food market have also started offering diet-friendly menu items.

> **Diet Alert**
>
> If you're on Weight Watchers, a medium serving of fries will set you back 6 points. Note also that for some fast-food items, the amount of digestible carbs goes over 100 grams, an amount that could be up to five times what you're allowed in a day. And some pre-packaged dressings might have 4 grams or more of digestible carbs per packet.

The pitfalls at these restaurants are legion, starting with white-bread buns and the French fries and continuing on through the sugary sauces and hydrogenated cooking oils.

Is it possible to eat in these restaurants and stick to your diet? Sure, but you'll need to have all your willpower about you. Pick from the salad portion of the menu, but beware of packaged dressings; they may pack on unwanted calories, carbs, and fat.

Plan ahead and bring a little jar of vinegar and oil dressing from home if you know you're going to order a salad.

For specific information on food at a particular restaurant, ask for a nutrition facts sheet; many of the fast food establishments now feature these brochures, and you can pick one up while you're waiting in line.

Delis

Oh, those wonderful places just around the corner with the to-die-for chicken salad and liverwurst sandwiches! Well, you don't have to swear off delicatessens altogether, but you do have to be smart about what you order. Cold cuts, even ones that are not fatty, tend to be high in sodium. If you're having problems losing weight and are having meals at the local deli, the sodium might be putting the brakes on your diet.

Soups without dumplings, vegetables, and simply prepared meats are the part of the menu you want to pay attention to. Be aware that the fat content on some of the prepared meats, such as pastrami, may tip you right out of your diet. Here's a twist for low-carb dieters: If you have a choice between low- or reduced-calorie dressings, take the high octane every time. Low-calorie dressings can have twice the digestible carbs in them that regular dressings do.

> **Diet Alert**
>
> If you're on a low-carb plan, the rye wheat bread that you think might be more "free" than white flour bread may be a surprise. Two slices of rye have 22 digestible carbs, which may be an entire day's limit that is spent on just one ingredient in one meal.

Alcohol

Whether you need your platinum credit card to take care of a restaurant bill or just that roll of quarters you had stashed away for an emergency, chances are the restaurant you opt for will have some kind of alcohol on the menu. All diet plans are concerned with chronic use of alcohol and deplore heavy use of it as inhibiting the healthy chemical reactions in the body that help you lose weight. On the other hand, nearly all diet experts say that drinking in moderation is fine, just don't overdo it.

If you like a glass with dinner, Ann Louise Gittleman, author of *The Fat Flush Plan*, suggests buying organic wines that are free of sulfites. Lower-end restaurants probably won't let you bring your own bottle, but higher-end restaurants often will charge a *corking fee*, and let you tote one in. If this is important to you, ask about this courtesy when you make your reservations.

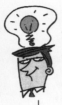

Tips to Use

What's moderation? Barry Sears, author of *The Zone*, says one glass of wine, preferably red, a day is a good limit.

Two major negatives to alcohol: Many experts say it interferes with how the liver works, and it weakens inhibitions. So, even if your liver is fine with alcohol, you still might be setting yourself up for a quick slide down a slippery slope; drinking makes saying yes to that slab of cheesecake so very easy. Alcohol can weaken your willpower, and if you want to lose weight, you must have all the discipline you can muster.

Let's talk specifics.

Wine

The debate over whether white wine is healthier than red wine is still as heated as it ever was. At the center of this argument is the *French paradox*. This is the seeming phenomenon whereby the French, even though they eat much more fat and have a superficially more heart-clogging diet than Americans do, have much less heart disease.

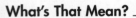

What's That Mean?

French paradox refers to the contradiction between the idea that the French diet, while much higher in saturated fat than an American diet, may cause fewer cancers and less death from heart disease. Many studies say this is because the French drink more wine than we do.

Studies have shown that certain chemicals in red wine may help protect the heart. Other studies have shown this same protective effect with white wine. Still others have shown it with grape juice. There is no definitive answer, but scientists and other researchers seem to agree that, unless you have a health problem that precludes your drinking wine, a glass now and then is probably good for your health. Another argument for a glass every now and then is that alcohol has a mild calming effect and can relieve a certain amount of stress. Because stress is at the core of many health problems, relieving it would help your health to some degree.

Beer

Beer and ale tend to be a heavy load when it comes to calories and carbohydrates, and you might want to forego the pleasure after you find out the effect they have on your diet.

If you're reading a book in 100-degree heat, pounding down a six-pack, and thinking you'll just sweat it all off, think again. You will likely find yourself at a weight loss stall. Here's how the U.S. Department of Agriculture stacks up the two main types of beer (for low-carb dieters, the carb count is "net"; the fiber has already been subtracted):

- Beer, ale, 1 can (12 fl. oz.): 146 calories, 12 carbs

- Lite beer, 1 can (12 fl. oz.): 99 calories, 5 carbs

Different brands of beer may have different carb and calorie counts, but the above numbers are a good starting point.

Hard Liquor

The concept of drinking in moderation certainly applies here.

A fluid ounce of, say, whiskey, goes a very long way toward making you feel more relaxed, easing stress, and all the other good things alcohol can do for you. Two fluid ounces may be taking a good thing just a little too far, however, and more than that at one time is probably not a good idea even if you have no health problems that preclude this amount.

Another problem with hard liquor is the tendency to mix it with colas, fruit juices, and other liquids. These mixers usually are sugary, so be prepared for quite a hit when you figure your carb or calorie count.

One fluid ounce of tequila, brandy, cognac, or vodka has no carbs, but each one of these liquors has 64 calories per fluid ounce. One

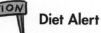

Diet Alert _____

Many hard liquors—vodka, for instance—have no carbs, but don't be lulled by a false sense of "free food" if you're on a low-carb diet. Hard liquors still have calories, and they still can affect your liver.

Check This Out

Because the liver figures heavily in metabolizing alcohol, and because that organ also is key in releasing and storing carbohydrates, a low-carb dieter might want to think twice before giving the liver double duty, even when the alcohol itself has few or no carbs.

fluid ounce of whiskey, bourbon, scotch, or rye also has no carbs, but will pack on 70 calories per fluid ounce.

The story with mixed drinks is slightly different. The calorie count goes down, but the carb count goes up. One fluid ounce of a tequila sunrise, for instance, has 34 calories and 3 digestible carbs. One fluid ounce of a whiskey sour, for example, has 41 calories plus 2 digestible carbs. Considering that these mixed drinks will generally come in 4 oz.—or much larger—glasses, these drinks can set the stage for a setback in your diet.

Beverages

Okay, so you've decided to skip the wine list and forego the mixed drink. What's left? Plenty. Although you might want to tread carefully here, too.

> **CAUTION**
> **Diet Alert**
> If you feel like a glass of milk, you may want to rethink your choice. Every degree of milk, from whole and 2 percent to nonfat skim, has 11 or more digestible carbs per cup and from 86 to 150 calories. Chocolate milk, of any degree of fat content, has 24 or more digestible carbs per cup and up to 208 calories.

Six fluid ounces of brewed black tea has only 1 digestible carb and 2 calories; the same amount of chamomile or any other herb tea has just 2 calories and only a trace amount of carbs.

If you're leaning toward soft drinks, stick to the diet varieties. For instance, a 12-ounce can of diet ginger ale has no carbs and no calories. Regular ginger ale, the same size can, has 32 digestible carbs and 124 calories. It's the same story with root beer: A can of diet root beer has no calories and no carbs; the regular has 39 digestible carbs and 152 calories. A can of a cola-type drink has 38 digestible carbs and 152 calories. The diet variety has only 4 calories and just a trace of carbohydrates.

Don't forget: Mineral water is just fine with dinner.

> **CAUTION**
> **Diet Alert**
> Just because coffee is basically a free ride when it comes to calories (4), carbs (1), and fat (a trace), don't get carried away. Starbucks' largest-sized White Chocolate Mocha coffee, made with half and half and topped with whipped cream, packs on 900 calories, 61 grams of fat, and 71 net carbs. A medium-sized skim latte is 160 calories, 0 fat, and 24 net carbs.

Running the Gantlet of Trigger Times

It's that holiday you can't possibly wiggle out of. It's the wedding or anniversary or business trip for which no excuse for not showing up will ever be good enough.

Accept the inevitable. You *will* be sitting at the Thanksgiving dinner table—or the Christmas one—or staring out over acres of food at office parties, business trips, or any one of dozens more occasions. That's the given. Your dilemma is not how to avoid these gatherings, but how to make it through them, your diet unscathed.

Check This Out

The good news is that you will probably gain less than 1 pound after the end-of-the-year holidays. This counters the popular belief that you will gain 5 pounds during the Christmas and New Year's season, says a small study done by researchers at the National Institute of Child Health and Human Development and the National Institute of Diabetes and Digestive and Kidney Diseases. Here's the bad news: That 1 pound stays with you, maybe for a lifetime. Also, if you're already overweight, you're more likely to gain those 5 pounds that everybody else only thinks they will.

Here are a few tips that may save your diet:

- **Eat something before you go.** Starving all day in anticipation will only sabotage you. A little soup or a bit of protein will help curb your appetite.

- **Stay across the room from the hors d'oeuvres or buffet table.** In fact, stand or sit with your back to it. You won't be tempted by what you can't see.

- **Eat slowly.** Give your stomach time to register what you've swallowed, and you'll want less.

- **Listen to your stomach.** When it's telling you it feels full, listen to it. Stop eating.

- **Fill your champagne or wine glass with sparkling water.** You'll still feel festive, but you won't blow your diet. You still might have enough room in your diet for a glass or two of wine, along with the water.

- **Don't forget: If you're the host or hostess, you get to choose the foods.** Choose foods that will allow you to stay on your diet, and don't worry that crazy Aunt Matilda will gossip about the lack of deep-fried hushpuppies, breaded shrimp, and buttery mashed potatoes. You might be surprised how many people would appreciate a healthy change of pace.

◆ **Refocus your attention.** A celebration can be about meeting new people, dancing, talking, and having fun. Think of food as the afterthought to the event, not the overriding theme that dwarfs all else.

Thanksgiving

Nothing says "groaning table" and "arise and waddle" the way that this November holiday does. There's no point in lamenting its evolution from a spiritual day of gratitude to a no-holds-barred major pig out and football fest. Your challenge is to deal with the reality and still keep to your diet.

Remember: Vegetables, normal portions, and no seconds should be your mantra here. A little slippage here and there is probably inevitable, but a forkful of pumpkin pie off of your spouse's plate is better than eating a whole piece. With ice cream. And whipped cream.

Christmas

Food seems to be everywhere during this holiday. Even Santa gets in on the act with his plate of cookies and milk. You might want to let Santa know that that medium-sized sugar cookie piles on 10 digestible carbs and 72 calories, and that cup of regular milk weighs in with 12 digestible carbs and 150 calories.

From early in the morning, when you're opening the presents, to later in the evening, watching still another rerun of *It's a Wonderful Life*, this holiday is packed with food. Even if you're strictly among your immediate family, it seems that food and munchies are at arm's length all day. Here's a hint for you: Stay more than arm's length away from all the bowls and plates of food. Proximity is an invitation to fall off of your diet.

Concentrate on eating raw vegetables and drinking plenty of water. You'll be amazed at how doing these two things will help you out.

New Year's

Drinking is probably the primary concern when you go out for a good time on New Year's Eve. Let's say you're going out to a restaurant for the evening.

Best thing to do: Eat something before you go out. Make your first drink water, and get out on the dance floor as soon as the music starts playing. Think about this: For every 20 minutes you're out on the dance floor, you're burning more than 100 calories. More importantly, you are most definitely not sitting at the table, eating and drinking everything in sight.

That takes care of New Year's Eve, but then you have New Year's Day, an endless round of football games, snacking, and visiting friends. Follow the advice we gave at the beginning of this chapter, and you'll make it through just fine.

> **Check This Out**
>
> Beer and wine tend to be heavier carb loads than hard liquor; wine tends to be the lightest calorie hit. But you're going to be pickled before midnight if you're hitting the vodka right from the start of the evening. Plan ahead as to what you will drink, follow your plan, and remember that the object of the evening is to have fun, not just to eat and drink.

> **Check This Out**
>
> What do some gravies, soft drinks, and baked goods have in common if you buy them from the supermarket? Chances are their caramel tint comes from a color additive made by heating sugar and other carbohydrates under controlled conditions. Especially if you're on a low-carb diet, this additive is definitely something you want to avoid.

Social Gatherings

Whether the invitation comes in the mail, over the phone, or by means of your second cousin once removed on your mother's side, the reaction is usually the same: fear.

For a dieter—birthdays, anniversaries, weddings, office parties, and other occasions usually mean total immersion in relatives, acquaintances, and other people you see only once a year. It also means resisting the cowardly urge to escape to the hors d'oeuvres or buffet table rather than struggle to remember what name goes with what vaguely familiar face. Whatever you do, don't take the cowardly way out. Advice in these situations echoes those words of wisdom for girding yourself before the holiday onslaught of temptation: Keep away from the tables of food and trays of nibbles. Try to keep to your regular schedule of meals, and don't starve yourself all day anticipating the after-event troughs of food. Be sensible, stick to your diet, and don't make the event about food; make it about the event.

The following sections provide tips to get you over the speed bumps with as little damage as possible.

Weddings

For a bride, the wedding is all about the dress; for a guest, it's all about the food. Get yourself out of that mentality and into another train of thought. For instance, take a camera along with you and snap candid photos of the guests and reception. Follow through on this by making an album of the photos and presenting it to the couple as an added wedding gift. They'll be thrilled because a professional photographer has a set repertoire of photos he takes (the bride's table, the toast, and so on), and there usually is not much leeway—or budget—for candid shots. It's important to tell the couple you're doing this because it commits you in a way that just snapping photos does not. It also keeps the camera in your hands instead of those deep-fried shrimp nibbles the waiters are passing out.

Don't forget to dance. Especially at weddings, you don't even need a partner; the floor is usually so crowded that no one even notices if there are partners or not. Even if your dancing ability is limited to flapping your arms and twirling, you'll still be speeding up your metabolism, and you won't be thinking about the dessert tray that's being passed around.

Birthdays and Anniversaries

These celebrations can be as simple as a family get-together or as elaborate as a major milestone event. If it's a simple family visit, you can ask your relative for sympathy; the host or hostess will probably be glad to arrange a meal that will fit in with your diet. If the event is more formal, you might not have the request option.

The real ordeal comes with serving the cake. It's almost impossible to wiggle out of a piece, but give it your best shot. If you can get past the cake, you're pretty much home free.

> **Tips to Use**
>
> Take a camera and tell your host you'll be making up a photo album for the lucky celebrants; this will keep your hands busy and out of the potato chips.

Office Parties

The boss is smiling, the caterers have just arrived, and the trays of food are being unveiled in the conference room. No matter what the reason for your office party—birthdays, an up-tick in sales, a promotion, or some other reason—an appearance at these functions is usually a smart idea. Bosses like to see the smiling faces of their happy employees, so show up and put your time in.

The trick with an office party is to remember that it's not particularly personal. If you don't show up on time, no one will notice, unless, of course, you're the boss. So don't show up on time. The best thing to do is to run into the room 15 minutes late, slightly breathless, and with apologies springing to your lips. Make it clear you were sacrificing your place at the giant hero sandwich in favor of taking care of important business that will be good for the company, so you can have even more giant hero sandwich parties in the future. By the time you get to the conference room, the food will have been ravaged, and it will be much easier to resist. If you're lucky, it will all be gone. A variation on this theme is to quietly arrive long after the party begins and ooze into the fringe of the gathering and stay there. When people ask where you've been, looked puzzled, look them in the eye, and tell them you've been there all along. It's amazing what people will believe if they have enough potato salad, bologna sand-wiches, and cookies on their plates to keep them occupied.

Business Trips

Any time you're away from home, it's going to be a challenge to stay on your diet. The rules of the road apply here. Bring a good supply of legal snacks and other foods you can have.

After you get to the hotel room, hand the key to the in-room snack locker back to the concierge. Getting rid of that key might save you a midnight raid when you're too wakeful to sleep and too bored for TV.

Diet Alert

Eggs, bacon, and cheese are not only encouraged on most low-carb diets, but they're the breakfast foods that are usually offered at the buffet at most hotels. The trick is to remember portion sizes and stop eating when you start to feel full.

During the day, when you have meetings or other business-related responsibilities, keeping on your diet may be easier than you think. Lunch will probably be at a restaurant, and fish or other legal foods will probably be on the menu. Drink mineral water, substitute vegetables for the rice or potato, and you're basically home free.

Dinner is usually when you're on your own, and you can keep to your diet easily when you don't have to compromise with anyone else.

I'm Tired, I'm Stressed—Where's the Potato Chips?

Screaming kids, inescapable boss, deadlines that just keep coming—even reading the words may make you want to bolt for the refrigerator and stuff yourself. Not only is this long-term chronic stress a common trigger for eating, it's also one that has a scientific reason behind it. When you're under short-term stress—say, someone cuts you off in traffic—the body has a feedback system that lets the adrenal stress system wind down. This is why you don't have to stop after every minor incident of road rage and relieve the stress with a large bag of French fries.

Check This Out
Scientists think that the adrenal stress system going into overdrive may be why people reach for the chocolate chip cookies and the greasy pizza when they are under constant stress.

But when stress just won't let up for days, weeks, or even months, the system in the body that deals with stress becomes chronically excited. The hormones unleashed by this state of chronic stress make the body want to engage in pleasurable activities. In a 2003 study of rats, animals under a constant state of stress over-ate high-energy comfort foods or became compulsive. The result: The rats got fat, especially in the abdominal area.

Tiredness

It's hard to talk about triggers for overeating without talking about tiredness. Think about it: When you're well rested, do you really feel as much pressure as when you're dog-tired? When you've had plenty of restful sleep, do you have the same urge to raid the refrigerator as when you're totally beat? Chances are the answer to both of those questions is no.

Tips to Use
Your tiredness might be your body telling you that you need to drink more water. Dehydration often shows up as fatigue.

Why should fatigue be a trigger? It takes energy and alertness to resist temptation, to keep to a discipline. When that energy is sapped, determination, discipline, and your diet tend to jump hand-in-hand right out the window.

Also, be sure you are not skipping meals or eating too little; both of these can be factors in how tired you feel. If you've been putting off starting your exercise program, get off of your chair and take a walk around the block. Your tiredness might be the result of a body that is not moving enough.

Stress

Stress actually has a purpose, and it served our ancestors well when they had to do things such as run away from wild boars that rampaged through their camps. If people were blasé about the boar, they'd be gored to death. The brain, however, developed a system of alerting the body and mustering up the energy to run. The brain starts a chain reaction that ends in stress hormones, such as *cortisol*, being released in the body. These stress hormones help turn blood sugar (glucose) and fatty acids into energy, so the muscles quickly have something to burn. After the crisis, the hormones are still high and make you feel hungry because the body wants that used energy to be replenished.

But what worked well for cavemen doesn't always work well in a society where dealing with waiting lines, jostling crowds, and jammed traffic while juggling career and family are almost a constant from dawn till dusk. If our stress is relatively constant, or even if it just spikes now and then, the stress hormones released will fuel the desire to eat (the body's mistaken attempt to replenish an energy that hasn't really been used).

The solution is to de-stress your life, which may be easier said than done. Instead of reaching for a cigarette, a drink, or a chocolate truffle, try the simplest thing first: Get out of your chair and walk. Exercise relieves stress, and you don't need to invest in equipment, elaborate workout clothes, or even an expensive gym membership.

What's That Mean?

Cortisol is a hormone made by the adrenal glands and is important in activating the immune system and processing carbohydrates. High amounts of it are released in moments of stress.

Tips to Use

A good yoga class is often only a channel surf away on the local PBS station. Offer to exercise your neighbor's dog; the neighbor will be grateful, the dog will be deliriously happy, and you'll be walking briskly to keep up.

Sleep Problems

One problem with being overweight is that it may cause problems sleeping. Sometimes, these problems spill over onto your family, and they have to bear the brunt of such noisy insomnia-creators as loud snoring. If you can never get a really sound sleep, you're going to feel tired most of the time. When you're tired, your willpower will be affected, and you'll have a harder time keeping to your diet.

Apnea

If you wake up in the morning with a headache and feel dead tired all day, it might be because you're not getting the kind of sleep you need. One common ailment that interrupts sleep is called *apnea*, from the Greek word meaning "want of breath." Either your brain is not sending the correct signals to the muscles that help you breathe, or your breath is constricted in some manner to where it can't flow properly. The latter kind, obstructive apnea, is far more common than the former type.

> **What's That Mean?**
>
> Apnea is a frequent disruption in sleep from blocked or constricted airflow caused by a physical obstruction in the upper airway or a missed signal from the brain to the respiratory muscles. It affects about 2.5 million of the 30 million Americans who snore.

If you think that merely waking up a lot—in some cases, 30 or more times an hour—doesn't really sound that bad, here's something to consider: Apnea is linked to irregular heartbeats, heart attacks, high blood pressure, and strokes.

If you suspect you might have this condition, or someone near to you tells you that you have the symptoms of apnea, see your doctor for a full evaluation.

Snoring

It sounds as though a tub full of bricks is rattling down the roof. That may be how snoring sounds to the one who falls asleep second. Even though it can be loud and annoying, nearly half of all normal adults snore every now and then; about 1 in 4 snore habitually. This is also a problem linked to being overweight, and it generally gets worse as you age.

Even though snoring might be annoying for those who have to listen to it, it's basically harmless.

How does this relate to your diet? Snoring can disrupt your sleep, and if your sleep is disrupted, you'll be tired the next day. If you're tired, your willpower goes down. When your willpower goes down, your diet suffers. All those foods you could resist when you were rested and felt good, are now all but on your plate and in your mouth.

You can help yourself to some extent. Stop drinking alcohol. Alcohol and some drugs make you sleepy, and, if you don't have good muscle tone in the tongue and throat, the tongue can fall to the back of the throat, or the muscles on the sides can draw in. Both events constrict the throat and cause snoring.

> **Check This Out**
>
> What causes snoring? Air can't flow freely through the passages at the back of the mouth and nose. This is the area where soft, flexible tissues are, and when the tongue, the uvula, and the soft palate meet, air is constricted, the tissues vibrate, and snoring results. Snoring can also be caused by a stuffy nose, which is why some people only snore during allergy season.

If you have large tonsils or adenoids or if you're overweight with a bulky neck, these can contribute to snoring.

Deformities inside the nose can also be the root of the problem. There are various treatments for snoring, and they range from wearing a special mask to surgery, but what is right for you will depend on what your doctor finds after an examination.

Do you have a sleep problem? Although it's impossible to diagnose anyone just by answering a few questions in a book, answering yes to many of the questions that follow may be grounds for calling your doctor for a thorough examination.

Sleep Inventory

Symptom	Yes	No
Do you snore so loudly that it wakes you up?	❑	❑
Are you usually tired during the day?	❑	❑
Do you nod off periodically during the day?	❑	❑
Have you been told you stop breathing momentarily during sleep?	❑	❑
Do you sometimes wake up with the sensation that you were choking?	❑	❑

continues

Sleep Inventory (continued)

Symptom	Yes	No
Do you sometimes wake up suddenly during the night and have to gasp for breath?	❑	❑
Do you have high blood pressure?	❑	❑
Are you irritable during the day?	❑	❑
Do you have morning headaches?	❑	❑
Do you have memory or concentration problems?	❑	❑
Is your throat dry when you wake up?	❑	❑

Cravings

If these mindless rampages through your cupboards make no sense to you, pay more attention to your daily food journal. Writing down how you feel, the stresses you are under, and other factors in your life might help you realize what is causing your craving. When you know the cause, you're halfway to knowing how to head it off.

Have plenty of legal snacks on hand for these times. Starving yourself is not going to solve the problem, and it may make your craving even more compelling.

Tips to Use

Even though we've said it before, it still bears repeating: Drink more water. Your body may be confusing dehydration with hunger. Have water beside you when you're working. Have a glass on the table next to you when you're watching television. It's a painless way to drink the water you need, and you'll hardly even know you've drunk your daily minimum until you check your journal.

Start Cooking

Chances are that, over the years, you fell into routines that involved grabbing something at the snack bar or local fast food place, or chugging something from soda machines (those extravaganzas of sugar and empty calories).

When you cook, you control everything that goes into your food, and you can keep on your plan a lot easier. It doesn't take monumental effort; many of the meal plans and recipes offered by the various diet authors can be prepared in literally minutes.

Make Meals Ahead of Time

Preparation is everything, and nowhere is that more true than in your diet. Making meals in bulk also keeps you from being chained to the stove. For instance, if you make meatloaf, divide it into portions after it's made and freeze each portion. You can do the same with most entrées, and you'll be set for the week—or longer.

And don't forget sauces. A good way to keep freshly made pesto, the Italian basil sauce that's good on everything from fish and pasta to chicken, is to make a batch, and then freeze it in portions in an ice cube tray. Each frozen cube can be one serving. After the sauce is frozen, store the cubes in a freezer bag and use them when you need them.

Keep Allowed Snacks Handy

This almost goes without saying, but a reminder never hurts: You're going to have some weak days where you'll want to eat everything in sight—prepare for them. The snacks you are allowed depend on which diet you're on and what stage you are at.

To prepare for a snack attack, you should eliminate the forbidden foods altogether from your kitchen. If it's not there, it's not going to tempt you.

Tips to Use

In the first, most strict phase of the low-carb Atkins diet, for example, you might want to keep on hand such things as deviled eggs and peeled shrimp for snacks. You can also have up to a quarter-pound of certain cheeses every day.

Brown Bag Your Lunch

The snack cart that rolls through the aisles, the cafeteria just down the hall that only ever seems to have sticky rolls left when you get your break, the vending machines that cough up 40 different kinds of packaged sugar—you might be forced to meet your enemy on its own territory, but there's one ultimate defense: Bring your own food.

To brown bag successfully, you should look to your youth. There were two rules of the elementary school blackboard jungle: Don't wolf what's in your bag on your way to school—you'll be starving all day—and always have a snack to tide you over.

You may be all grown up, but the rules still apply. Don't eat your lunch until your actual lunch time.

Packing your lunch is also a lot cheaper than grazing all day off the snack cart, and here's a way to reward yourself for your frugality and self-discipline: Figure out how much money you were spending on food at work before your diet, and figure out how much your brown bag lunch costs you. Subtract the two figures, and use the money you are saving yourself to buy a treat. And make it a good one: a new pair of hockey skates, a full day of pampering at the spa, two tickets to the playoff game, or any other pleasurable goal you always kind of wanted but never really wanted to spend the money on. Now you'll have the money, and you'll look great, as well.

Tips to Use

Make sure you have a snack for those low-energy moments that usually happen around mid-morning and mid-afternoon. Your snacks will take the edge off and help keep your discipline in good shape.

Trash Fattening Foods

We know, we know. Mom always said that throwing away food is a waste, but sometimes keeping it is a bigger waste—that goes right to your waist.

Deep six that 5-pound bag of sugar; dump those candy bars you've hidden in the meat compartment of the fridge; put your foot on that bag of potato chips and sprinkle the crumbs into the garbage can. Say aloha to the foods that are not your friends.

Canned goods are a different story. Contribute the unopened cans of forbidden food to a local food bank. Just because you don't want them doesn't mean no one else wants them. You may even get a tax break.

Enlist Your Family

This may be the biggest aid of all. If your spouse, your children, and the other people closest to you wish you well, you're halfway to your goal.

Right from the beginning, involve your family. Sit everyone down at the kitchen table and tell them how you feel, how being fat makes you feel, how you're worried about your health, and, most importantly, how you really need their help. Even the most surly, tattooed, pierced, and rebellious teenager will answer a plea like that.

Just be prepared to accept the help, which is the other end of the bargain. After you ask for their help, it's your job to say yes when they ask you to go for a walk around the block. It is your job to say yes when they want some help gathering up fallen branches, mowing the lawn, or going with them to a school or work event. You are going on a diet to change your life; don't drag your feet when your life actually starts to change. Say yes to everything. Except food.

Diet Alert

Beware of subtle sabotage. One woman had lost more than 20 pounds and was regaining a sense of confidence and sexiness. Her husband, all the while protesting his support, went out and bought a $250 deep fat fryer. Sabotage? The woman thought so and wrapped the fryer in a plastic garbage bag and let it melt in the attic over a few hot summers.

Have a Plan

The world doesn't stop because you're on a diet. Pets will die, your kid's grades will nosedive, your mother-in-law will come to live with you—the list of potential problems is endless. The way you handle these problems will determine if your diet will be successful.

Many crises will be bolts from the blue, and you will not be able to prepare for them. Others can be prepared for down to the last minute. One way of girding your mental loins for these challenges is by knowing exactly what knocks you off your diet. The following form will help you pinpoint your trouble spots. Fill in the Event blank with something that stresses you, for instance, "tax time." In the next blanks, write down foods and drinks you can consume and those you should avoid to stave off a binge. Write down what drives you crazy, for instance, "I have to hunt down tax receipts," and how you can get past this stress. For instance, write in "having all my folders on the desk in advance." Make as many copies of this form as you need to.

Event Checklist

Event: _____

Foods I can eat (and how much): _____

_____

_____

Foods to avoid: _____

_____

_____

What I can drink: _____

_____

It always drives me crazy when: _____

_____

I can get past my crazy makers by: _____

_____

_____

The Least You Need to Know

- ◆ Events that trigger binges are inevitable, but planning ahead will help get you through them.

- ◆ Long-term stress can change your body chemistry in ways that can throw you off your diet.

- ◆ Sleep problems can sabotage your diet.

- ◆ Enlisting your family and friends will help you succeed in losing weight.

- ◆ Keeping a daily journal will help pinpoint problems and help you find solutions.

Chapter 4

Work It Out and Work It Off

In This Chapter

- ◆ Working out the easy way
- ◆ Walking off the pounds
- ◆ Figuring out how fast your metabolism is
- ◆ Achieving great results with little effort: pushups and squats

Exercise is one aspect of dieting where all the experts agree: Start moving your body, getting your blood pumping harder, and strengthening your muscles. This is a triumvirate of activity that will normally suppress your appetite, help you to lose weight, and keep you on your diet. And you don't need a vein-popping, sweat-dripping workout to achieve all these benefits. Even a mild workout will go a long way toward strengthening your body. Taking a walk is easy, and that's always a good place to start.

In this chapter, you'll find out what experts recommend making part of your workout—and you might be surprised at what they suggest. You'll also learn that intensity may not be the boon you figured it to be and why easy-does-it might do the job just as well.

You'll discover how to do the recommended exercises in a safe way. You'll also find out how fast your heart should be beating during exercise and what the least amount of energy is that you need to sustain your body, by simply filling in some short forms.

Diet Alert

Never start any exercise program without talking to your doctor first.

You'll learn what activities are moderate or difficult, how many calories they make you burn in a set amount of time, and how to work your way up slowly to a good, solid general workout.

And, Yes, Talk to Your Doctor

Especially if you have been inactive for a long time, it's essential to talk to your doctor before you pound around in an aerobics class at the gym, drop into that kung fu course you have been intending to take, or jump on your bike and pedal 20 miles.

You might also want to take a look at various exercises and the calories they burn; the following table lists calories expended by a 150-pound person exercising for 20 minutes and might give you some ideas as to what you would like to do.

Exercises and the Calories They Burn

Exercise	Intensity	Calories Used
Volleyball	Moderate	70
Walking 3 mph	Moderate	81
Walking 4 mph	Moderate	94
Jogging 5 mph	Hard	167
Running 6 mph	Very Hard	231
Ping-pong	Moderate	94
Raking leaves	Moderate	94
Social dancing	Moderate	103
Mowing lawn w/power mower	Moderate	103
Field hockey	Hard	188

Source: Surgeon General's Report on Physical Activity and Health, 1996

If you're under 35 and healthy, you probably don't have much to worry about—but it's still good to see your doctor; he's in a good position to recommend what kind of exercise program you should be on. If you're over 35, your doctor may want to do a few tests to see what your heart and endurance are like.

You'll most certainly want to get medical clearance if you have any of the following conditions:

- High blood pressure
- Heart problems
- Family history of stroke or heart attacks
- Dizzy spells
- Extreme breathlessness after even slight exertion
- Arthritis or bone problems
- Extreme muscle or connective tissue problems
- Any other disease you know you have

Take a Walk

Every diet touts the many benefits of simply strapping on a pair of comfy shoes and going for a walk. This simple exercise is underrated by people who think you have to feel the burn and drip sweat to get into real shape. But that no-pain-no-gain attitude is falling by the wayside as more research shows that walking will not only help you lose weight, but it is also linked to a lower rate of heart disease.

Not only will you look better and your clothes will fit better, but the changes go all the way to the core. Your internal organs will work better, and your blood vessels, muscles, and heart will be more efficient.

Exercise also helps if you're watching carbs—your insulin levels will probably stabilize or even go down, an effect central to a low-carb diet's success.

Keep in mind that a real walk is not simply a stroll to the soft drink vending machine. You'll want to move at a brisk and steady enough clip to make your heart beat faster and make you breathe more deeply.

> **Check This Out**
>
> A 2003 study supported by the National Heart, Lung, and Blood Institute showed that walking briskly worked just as well as a more intense workout when it came to losing weight—and keeping it off.

A good way of telling if you're getting the best out of your exercise is to figure out if your heart is beating within a range that makes the most of the activity. To figure out if you're exercising within these ranges, stop exercising briefly and take your pulse. Your heart should beat within your optimal range for at least 20 minutes of your exercise routine.

Join the walkers of the world, and you join a dedicated group. Walking is the only exercise people keep up even into middle age and beyond. People usually drop out of other types of exercise, but they continue walking. In fact, the highest percentage (nearly 40 percent) of regular walkers is among men 65 and older.

Tips to Use

You can take your pulse at your neck, but the easiest way is to take it at your wrist. Put the tips of your index and middle fingers on the artery that travels along the wrist in a line with the thumb. Count the beats for a full 60 seconds, or count for 30 seconds and multiply by two. Start your count on a beat, and count that one as zero.

To find out your personal ranges for your target heart rate, fill in the following form and refer to it before you go out to exercise. You need to calculate your maximum heart rate for your age and then take a percentage of it to find out the best range for the activity you're doing. Your target heart rate should be 50 percent to 70 percent of your maximum heart rate if you're doing moderate exercise. For vigorous exercise, your range is 70 percent to 95 percent of your maximum heart rate.

Target Heart Rate

220 – _____ (my age) = _____ (max heart rate, beats per minute)

Moderate-Intensity Activity

Lower limit:
(max heart rate) _____ × 0.5 = _____ beats per minute
Upper limit:
(max heart rate) _____ × 0.7 = _____ beats per minute

Vigorous-Intensity Activity

Lower limit:
(max heart rate) _____ × 0.7 = _____ beats per minute
Upper limit:
(max heart rate) _____ × 0.85 = _____ beats per minute

Here's an example: Let's take a healthy 40-year-old man. Subtract his age from 220, and you get his maximum heart rate for his age. In this case, that number is 180. In your own case, you want to try not going over your own personal number of beats per minute when you exercise; prolonged stress on your heart might damage it.

Continuing the example, the man's lower limit for moderate exercise would be 180 × 0.5 = 90. His upper limit would be 180 × 0.7 = 126. So if the man in our example decided to walk briskly, he would have to keep his heart beating faster than 90 bpm but slower than 126 bpm for 20 minutes to get the most out of the exercise.

Don't Go Overboard

Here are the first three rules of beginning an exercise program:

- ◆ Patience
- ◆ Patience
- ◆ Patience

Start slowly after you've talked to your doctor and decided how much you can safely do, especially at first. Some experts say it might take a month or more to make up for each year you've been physically inactive. This means, if you've been a couch potato for six years, it may take you six months to build up your stamina and strength to an acceptable level.

In the beginning, experiment to see how far and fast you can walk without overdoing it. Start with a few minutes and add five minutes a week until you get up to 20 minutes or so four to five times a week. If you've been sedentary for a long time, you might want to start with just a minute or two. Rest a minute, and then walk a minute or two, repeating this walk-rest cycle until you are tired. As you continue your walking routine, you'll extend your distance and time and pick up your pace until you are walking briskly for about 30 minutes most days of the week.

The most important thing is to listen to your body and pay attention to what it's saying. If you get dizzy, have pain or nausea, or experience any other unusual symptom, either slow down or stop. See your doctor if the symptoms persist.

Tips to Use

What's the right pace? If you can walk and carry on a conversation, you're probably about right. If you're too breathless to talk, then you're probably going too fast.

The Beauty of Pushups and Squats

If walking begins the *aerobic* portion of your exercise program—the sort of exercise that requires oxygen—you should also think about beginning the *anaerobic* part. This is where you concentrate on building strength by exercising with weight. You don't have to invest a small fortune in gym memberships and coordinating outfits to get started on your weight-training program. In fact, the two basic exercises that will get you started rely solely on your own body weight to build your strength.

What's That Mean?

Aerobic literally means *with oxygen*, but when it comes to exercise, it means using major muscles to keep doing an activity for at least 15 minutes at a pace that is at least 60 percent of your maximum heart rate.

Anaerobic means *without oxygen*. This refers to exercise done by muscles at a high intensity for a short period of time.

Diet Alert

If you feel any pain at any time, stop what you're doing. Ask a trainer at your gym to watch as you do the exercise; you might be doing something wrong and not realize it. Correct positioning in weight training is essential.

You can start with the old reliables: pushups and squats. Before you roll your eyes and throw up your hands, consider their virtues. They take no special equipment, you can do them virtually anywhere, and you can—and should—begin doing them with gentleness and respect. You are not in Marine boot camp; if you could drop and do 20 pushups on command, you are already in good shape.

If your body is not strong enough to do a classic pushup, begin by standing near a wall, lean into it, and then push yourself away. When you can do 30 to 45 of these divided into three sets, then go to the next level, which is pushing away from a counter. Put your hands on a counter, and back your feet away from it a couple of feet. Lower your body with your hands, and then push it up again. Again, when you can do 30 to 45 of these divided into three sets, go to the next level, which are knee pushups. These are just like classic pushups, only your knees are the pivot point, not your feet. After you are strong enough to do the same repetitions you did for the easier two types of pushups, try the classic pushup. Always remember to keep your back straight and your abdominal muscles strong.

Squats have a controversial history, with some experts saying that these deep knee bends are bad for your knees, and other people swearing that if you do them correctly, they are the best thing in the world for working your lower body. Science comes down on the side of doing a shallow squat, not a deep knee bend, because the strain of the more extreme exercise might damage the *ligaments*.

Stand with your feet shoulder-width apart, your arms outstretched in front of you at shoulder level, and bend your knees gently and only as far as you feel comfortable. Also, be careful that your knees don't move past your toes, or, if they do, they don't move very far past them. Again, listen closely to your body; if your knees protest, then either don't do the exercise or squat less deeply.

You only need to do 5 or 10 minutes a day of this kind of strength training to start to build up your body. And remember what the three rules of beginning your exercise program are—patience, patience, patience!

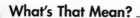

What's That Mean?

Ligaments are cord-like tissues that connect bones to other bones or to cartilage. They stabilize joints.

Increasing Your Workout Time

When you first begin your workout program, you may only be able to do a few minutes. Before you start feeling frustrated that you can't run the 400-yard dash or do 50 chin-ups in 1 minute, remember how long it took you to get in the shape you are now in. Be kind to your body, and it will respond to you.

Whatever your workout time is in the beginning, try to add a minute each day. Try to add at least 5 minutes each week until you are up to 30 minutes a day. After you are up to 30 minutes, you can start adding activities, start doing your exercises more intensely, and start having fun with your body—instead of always feeling you are fighting it.

Tips to Use

It's going to take you a while to tune up your body. Always keep in mind that you will eventually get where you are going if you take one measured step at a time and don't force your muscles to react.

The Argument for Lifting Weights

Many experts mention some kind of weight training as a good thing to do, not only to balance your exercise and the way your body is being toned, but also because it will build strength and add muscle in ways that strictly aerobic exercise (such as jogging or using a stair climbing machine in the gym) won't. If you have any kind of medical condition, ask your doctor if lifting weights is right for you. If you shouldn't do it, there is likely another kind of resistance training you can do and that your doctor can recommend.

Weight lifting or some kind of strength training also lets the body better use the insulin it makes, an essential element for a low-carb dieter. Using existing insulin is important in people whose cells become insensitive to insulin, triggering ever-increasing amounts of the hormone to do the basic job of normalizing blood sugar.

Strengthening your muscles has many benefits:

Diet Alert

Also, before working with weights, it's good to take a 5- or 10-minute walk to warm up your muscles. You're more likely to hurt yourself if you use weights without warming up your muscles.

- ◆ Your balance and coordination improve.
- ◆ You lift things more easily.
- ◆ Your bones become denser.
- ◆ You become less prone to injury.
- ◆ You feel more self-confident.
- ◆ Your metabolism speeds up.

Muscle burns three times more calories than fat does. In other words, even when you're sitting in a chair watching television, your muscles are burning up energy much faster than the fat cells in your body. The more muscle tissue you have, the more energy you're burning. The more energy you burn, the faster you'll lose weight.

What's That Mean?

Basal metabolic rate (BMR) is measured in calories and tells you how much energy is required to keep the body working when it is at rest.

About 70 percent of the energy you expend each day is what it takes to keep your lungs breathing, your heart beating, your temperature at a steady level, and your ability to maintain other basic functions of life. This energy level is called the *basal metabolic rate (BMR)*. If you know your BMR, you know the least number of calories you need to keep your body functioning.

The following table gives you the formula for figuring out your BMR. Fill in you BMR on the blank line in the table.

Calculate Your Basal Metabolism Rate

Age	Formula
	Men
18–30	6.95 × body weight + 679
30–60	5.27 × body weight + 879

Age	Formula
	Women
18–30	6.68 × body weight + 496
30–60	3.95 × body weight + 829

My BMR is _____ calories per day.

When you first begin to train and start to build some muscle mass, don't be surprised to see the scale nudge upward. Don't worry about this gain; you're acquiring muscle, and it's denser than fat. The same volume of muscle weighs more than the same volume of fat. Think of it this way: a box of nails weighs more than the same size box of feathers. Instead of letting the scale tell you how you're doing, ask yourself this: Do your clothes fit better? If the answer is yes, then you're doing fine.

Again, the objective is to start slowly so you don't injure yourself. If you belong to a gym, ask one of the staff trainers to design a program for you and have him or her go through the routine with you so that you always maintain the correct position whenever you lift weights.

If you don't belong to a gym, take the low-tech approach. Use lightweight canned food for hand weights. Again, start slowly, and if you feel any pain, stop immediately and ask a professional to evaluate how you're doing the exercise.

> **Check This Out**
>
> Some women worry that weight training will bulk up their muscles like a man's. That's not likely. Women don't produce enough testosterone, the hormone abundant in men that is responsible for allowing men to build big muscles.

Ten Tips for Keeping Your Exercise Program on Track

After you start exercising, there might come a day when you sit back, roll your eyes skyward, and dread the start of your exercise routine. It's at this very point that you should forge ahead. Here are some ideas for getting past the exercise ennui:

- ◆ **Make a commitment.** Put it in writing, and tack it up where you can see it every day as a reminder. Consistency is everything in exercise; you must do it regularly to get the most benefit.

- ◆ **Fill out the exercise portion of your journal every day.** This accountability will help get you out of your chair and into your exercise.

- ◆ **Find an excuse to walk.** Take the stairs, not the elevator; park at the back of the lot, not the space closest the door; do mini-exercises at your desk. It all counts, and you may wind up doing more exercise than you ever thought.

- ◆ **Rediscover dancing.** Forget the I-can't-dance excuses; this is the perfect time for taking those tango lessons you always promised yourself. Or waltz. Or tap. And if you need a little incentive to overcome your shyness, just ask yourself this: Ever seen a fat tango dancer?

- ◆ **Exercise in the right shoes.** If you don't have the support, your feet will suffer. Ask a seasoned trainer at your gym for a recommendation.

- ◆ **Mini-lessons on the TV.** Don't underestimate the power of the tube. For a change of pace, tune in to any number of exercise programs, from yoga to famous-name fitness shows. Just make sure the show is at your level; when in doubt, opt for the slower, easier program until you become used to the routine. A little variety in your program will reinvigorate you.

- ◆ **Lower your expectations.** The desire for instant gratification can lead to injury. If you try to do too much too soon, you may damage your ligaments and joints, and this could set you back weeks.

- ◆ **Avoid injuries.** Always warm up and stretch before you exercise, and always go through your cool-down routine afterward. Both phases will help you avoid injury.

- ◆ **Don't buy into your own excuses.** You *do* have the time; staying fit doesn't have to be expensive; everyone is *not* looking at you; and exercising is *not* making you gain weight.

- ◆ **Have fun.** If you used to be the ping-pong champ of the eighth grade, rediscover the sport that made you feel so good. Or discover a new one.

The exercise portion of your diet can help you rediscover not only the fitness of your youth, but the joy you had in your body when you were a kid and cleaning your plate was the high price your mother exacted for going outside to play. Think of your exercise program not as one more thing you have to crowd into your day, but as your playtime. The more fun you have, the more likely you are to continue with your exercise, and the less likely you are to watch the clock while you are doing it. Just remember to go slowly and have patience, patience, patience.

The Least You Need to Know

- ◆ Exercise is an essential part of your diet.

- ◆ Start slowly and be patient with yourself.

- ◆ Low-tech exercising such as walking and doing pushups and squats are a good way to start.

- ◆ Increase the time and intensity of your exercise every day until you reach your optimum routine.

- ◆ Be meticulous about keeping your diet and exercise journal; it will motivate you and help you get where you're going.

Chapter 5

Leaping the Mental Hurdles

In This Chapter

- Opening social doors through weight loss
- Flirting might be intimidating
- Feeling confused about weight loss
- Rediscovering your inspiration

The mind often lags behind the body in adjusting to weight loss. People may have either ignored you or regarded you with the same interest they have for wallpaper; now, they may be looking at you with more sexual intent. As your weight changes, your role in society may also change (which could be disconcerting). In this chapter, you'll fill out a diary that will let you keep track of how other people are reacting to you, and how these reactions are affecting you. You'll also fill out a form where frankness and candor are the keys that will get you to the next level of weight loss and give you insight into how you really feel about losing weight.

You'll find many stumbling blocks can hold up your weight loss, but you'll also find solutions to many of these problems.

Why Do I Feel Confused?

Old friends never swung you off your feet when they first saw you; people didn't sit next to you on the bus because you spilled over into the next seat; you always needed to buy two airplane tickets; no one could ever hug you because they couldn't get their arms around you; you shopped for clothes alone so no one would see the double-digit sizes you bought; mirrors were the enemy. Now all that's changed since you've been losing weight, right? You've heard through the office grapevine that the dream down the hallway would really like to go out with you. When you look in the mirror, you're still surprised to see someone healthy—and just this side of unrecognizable—staring back at you. You feel bones you never felt before. People flirt with you. You can walk up a flight of stairs and not even breathe hard. Strangers strike up conversations with you. For the first time in your life, you're actually, well, *popular*. Losing weight is just like the picture you had in your head, isn't it?

Well, except for the fear part.

When you're standing on the cusp between your old heavyweight self and a newer, lighter weight version, there's bound to be some measure of internal confusion. People have reacted to you one way for probably most of your life, and now they are reacting to you in what is probably a very different way. And it is a way that carries you into a new arena of emotional responsibilities.

Adding in the Flirtation Factor

Whenever a handsome man or beautiful woman spoke to you before, it was only to ask if you could introduce them to your gorgeous, thin friend. Now, you *are* that gorgeous, thin friend, and others are making the introductions. Your social skills may not have evolved fast enough to absorb this kind of change. Hence, the fear factor.

One woman who lost more than 100 pounds described this stage of weight loss as being a time to contemplate a future that is both exciting and scary. Even though you may tell yourself how much you hate that layer of fat that separates you from the world, the fact is that layer of fat is familiar, and losing it is leaving behind the life you've known for something unfamiliar and full of frightening expectations.

It might take you a while to re-learn how to talk to the opposite sex. You might want to prime the pump a bit by reading the rapier wits and lyrical romantics of times gone by. Check out British poet and playwright Oscar Wilde; American writer and satirist Dorothy Parker; and the ultimate in romantic poets, Elizabeth Barrett and Robert Browning. A nicely turned phrase is so rare in this world of slang, brutalized verbs, and anemic assertion that a well-placed snippet of a quote will mark you as educated and charming.

You might need a roadmap to see where your emotions are headed. The following form will help you figure out people's reactions and put them into perspective. We've divided the form into Friends, Family, Strangers, and Acquaintances because each of these groups will have a slightly different view of you. Under the category Who?, fill in either the person's name or some other identifying characteristic ("barista at coffee shop," and so on) that will jog your memory when you read this back to yourself weeks from now. Fill in the date and what was said. Under Uncomfortable Moments, cite the events that made you feel that way. Under Surprises, list the incidents or comments that came out of the blue and astonished you. Then record how all this made you feel. Crystallizing these feelings into words will help you cope with the changes you are undergoing.

> **Check This Out**
>
> Flirting is a system of signaling that is nature's way of letting you know who you should be going home with. The process seems to bypass all that is rational in the brain and dig down into behavior that is ruled by the most ancient parts of the brain—the impulsive parts that are most like those of animals.

> **Tips to Use**
>
> If you're nervous around the opposite sex, a bit of role playing may help. Imagine you're an actor, preparing for a role. Only this role is meeting someone new and making conversation. Visualize the encounter and what you'll say. This "rehearsal" will give you confidence when the real moment comes.

How People React to the New Me

Who?	Date	Compliments	Uncomfortable Moments	Surprises	How I Felt
Friends	___	_____	_____	_____	_____
_____	___	_____	_____	_____	_____
_____	___	_____	_____	_____	_____
_____	___	_____	_____	_____	_____
_____	___	_____	_____	_____	_____
_____	___	_____	_____	_____	_____
_____	___	_____	_____	_____	_____
_____	___	_____	_____	_____	_____
Family	___	_____	_____	_____	_____
_____	___	_____	_____	_____	_____
_____	___	_____	_____	_____	_____
_____	___	_____	_____	_____	_____
_____	___	_____	_____	_____	_____
_____	___	_____	_____	_____	_____
_____	___	_____	_____	_____	_____
Strangers	___	_____	_____	_____	_____
_____	___	_____	_____	_____	_____
_____	___	_____	_____	_____	_____
_____	___	_____	_____	_____	_____
_____	___	_____	_____	_____	_____
_____	___	_____	_____	_____	_____
_____	___	_____	_____	_____	_____

Who?	Date	Compliments	Uncomfortable Moments	Surprises	How I Felt
Acquaintances	___	___	___	___	___
___	___	___	___	___	___
___	___	___	___	___	___
___	___	___	___	___	___
___	___	___	___	___	___
___	___	___	___	___	___
___	___	___	___	___	___
___	___	___	___	___	___

Goodbye, Comfort Layer of Fat

As you get thinner, the physical layer that exists between you and other people is disappearing. You may have thought this is exactly what you wanted your entire life, but now that it is becoming a reality, you may feel something surprising: fright. You may head for the restroom when you see someone coming toward you who wants to go out with you. You may resist that big hug from the delighted someone who, for the first time, really does want to hug you. You may turn down opportunities to go out socially.

Tips to Use _____

Here's the easiest way in the world to give yourself a confident start to the day: Make the last thing in your morning bathroom routine a big, toothy grin. Smile at yourself in the mirror as though you're walking down the red carpet on your way to accepting an Oscar. You'll be surprised at how that image of happiness will follow you throughout the day.

When you lose a great deal of weight, attention begins to focus and gain momentum after you've lost about 35 pounds. The compliments and comments about your weight loss start coming regularly. The problem: To go from being virtually ignored to being admired may be a jolt for some people.

This jolt may rock you right off your diet. Somewhere inside you may want that comforting cover of fat again. If you've leveled out and can't figure out what's wrong, take a cool appraisal of yourself, and confront the feelings that may be holding you back. And don't forget about anger. Think about all those years when no one paid attention to you—does it now make you angry that people suddenly *are* paying attention to you? Does it make you angry that people couldn't see beyond the fat before? Does it make you angry that you are the same person now that you were before, but no one bothered to look?

Tips to Use

If you are angry, consider this possibility: You're *not* the same person you were when you were fat. You have acquired discipline, and you are probably fitter, healthier, and happier than you were when your world revolved around food. Your self-esteem probably rises every time you shop for clothes. Give other people a break; who wouldn't want to be around someone who is happier, more active, and more confident?

Fill out the following form with the idea that no one will ever read it except you. Be honest with yourself, and take a good, hard look at how you really feel. Having to put your thoughts down in writing may clarify issues that are deeply embedded and stopping you from getting below a certain level of weight.

How I Really Feel About Losing Weight

I love losing weight because it makes me feel ...

_____

_____

_____

_____

_____

_____

_____

_____

I don't like dieting because ...

_____

_____

_____

_____

_____

_____

_____

_____

I'm afraid of losing weight because ...

_____

_____

_____

_____

_____

_____

_____

_____

The Ho-Hum Factor

Nearly every dieter starts with high expectations, great discipline, and their heels firmly dug into the dieting landscape. After months of being "good," though, and never, ever going off your plan, it's almost inevitable that a bit of boredom creeps in. This is a common reason cited by dieters for veering off of their plan and into the world of forbidden foods and gargantuan portions.

If you veer too far off of your plan for too long, however, you may find yourself creeping back up into that Neverland of weight gain where returning to the discipline of your plan becomes harder and harder.

If you catch yourself being bored with your diet, there are probably several things at play. You could be eating too much of the same foods, day in and day out (even the most rigid and controlled diet plans encourage variety and experimentation with food).

The first thing to do is re-examine the foods you've crossed off your list. It's okay to put a *little* of just about anything back into your diet; you just can't put *a lot*. And a little of something you love can add enough spice in your diet to keep you motivated.

The second thing to do is to turn to your diet plan's menu and recipe section. Nearly every diet plan has back-of-the-book recipes or offers separate books that have menu plans and cooking tips. Make a date with yourself to cook at least one recommended meal every few days. Pick out foods you've never had before, and make them. You might be surprised how broad your culinary tastes become. You can also add interest to you diet by adding more vegetables or varying your snacks.

Another trick is to invite someone over for lunch or dinner. This forces a kind of formality on you that you may not have when it's just you or your immediate family. Preparing a real sit-down meal is a creative experience. Share it, and enjoy it. If you know other dieters, this could be a way to start a daisy chain of socialization. Have fun and get to know people while you are keeping to your diet.

> **Check This Out**
>
> Maybe you simply don't eat carb- and calorie-heavy pasta anymore. Which means, anything to do with pasta—sauces, for instance—automatically went down into the same black hole. Although commercial tomato sauces are fairly calorie friendly, they usually have a lot of carbs. Pesto sauce is good on low-carb diets, and this basil-based sauce is wonderful on chicken, fish, and other foods.

> ### Check This Out
>
> Don't forget about nuts if you're on a low-carb diet. You just have to be careful of the different varieties and watch how much of them you eat. Pecans, for instance, are a low-carb bargain (1.3 digestible carbs per ounce), while cashews (8.1 digestible carbs per ounce) are high enough to tip you out of your plan if you dip your hand in the bowl once too often.

Winning the Mental Game

Ask anyone who's fabulously successful, 9 out of 10 of them will tell you they don't have that much more talent or intelligence than anyone else. But what every single one of them will also tell you is that they had a million times more *desire* to succeed than anybody else. And that's the mental part of the process. You can lose weight and keep on losing it until you get to your goal, but unless you conquer the longing to slack off, to just not do it anymore, you'll be letting your goal slip between your fingers.

Don't let it.

Remember Your Goals and Dreams

The first time you feel the faintest flutter of surrender, take action fast. Go to your daily journal and re-read the entries you made from the very beginning of your diet. Oftentimes, just reading how you felt when the pounds were first coming off is enough to relive the joy of accomplishment, re-sparking your incentive.

When you first started your diet, you had certain goals: looking better and feeling better. But did you also want to be more personable, more popular, more desired by the opposite sex? Well, who wouldn't? The question to ask yourself when you're tempted to chuck your diet is, "Do I feel better now than I did before I went on my diet?" And by "feel better," we don't mean listing all the negatives you can think of: craving food, hating to limit portions, and all the other daily minutiae of dieting. We mean, do you really feel better? Do you like yourself more? Do others respond to you more? Do you have more self-respect? Do you have more confidence? Do you feel more in control of your life?

These are the feelings you should dwell on. These confidence builders will only get stronger as you continue to lose weight.

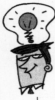

Keeping your daily journal is a way of recording all the various stages you go through. If you're feeling down about your diet and how you're doing on it, writing down your feelings may help clarify for you why you're feeling this way.

Get It in Writing

Make a list of the things that have gotten better in your life since you started your diet. Even if it sounds trivial, list it anyway.

It is only from experience that people grow. When you see how far you've come, it's easier to look ahead and see the opportunities instead of the potholes, quagmires, and traps that may lie around the bend. Because, guess what, all those stumbling blocks may not even exist, and you are talking yourself out of your goals if all you see are obstacles.

Consider a Therapist

Don't dismiss this suggestion out of hand. Even the strongest people can feel a quiver at the knees.

Also, be prepared for reactions from other people that you may not expect. Family members may resent your refocused attention. Friends may drift away or say they liked the "old you" better. In the face of all these pressures to go back to being "good old you," you may feel like giving in and doing what everyone else seems to want.

Tips to Use

If you see a therapist, you may discover that the people around you had a point: You were veering a bit too extremely, and you should come back into the orbit of your friends and family a little more.

Don't.

You have a period of adjustment, but so will most of the people in your life. If this period is not resolving itself happily, sit those people down and have a frank talk with them about how much losing weight means to you. Even if they nod and smile and say they understand, you may also want to take it one step further and get some professional help. Involving an impartial third party often clarifies *everyone's* position.

Re-read Your Diet Book—and Others

After you've been on your plan for a while, you'll probably be referring to its pages less and less. The day will come when you will shut it completely and put it back up on the bookshelf whence it came.

That's fine. You may know your diet so well that you no longer need a 300-page reminder lying around the kitchen. What many people find, though, is that a day comes when they realize they're bored to tears with their diet, they're sick of all the counting, counting, counting, and that chunk of cheesecake down at the deli isn't looking so bad, after all. It's at this point that you should slap your hands away from the refrigerator and get that diet book back down from the shelf. Approach the book as something new, something you haven't read before. Start at the beginning and read all the inspiring stories of people who have lost weight, reveling in the joy they feel about how their lives have changed.

It's a way of reliving that initial rush of enthusiasm for your plan. Yet another way is to take a look at some other diet books. Take one or two out of the library; this detour doesn't have to be expensive. As you read other books and the different philosophies of their authors, you might pick up a few tips and become energized once again.

> **Tips to Use**
>
> Long-time dieters tend to cherry-pick items from other diets. Many times they wind up with their own customized plan for losing weight, cobbled together from many other plans and authors.

You can win the mental game.

The Least You Need to Know

- As you lose weight, you may have to adjust for people's changing reactions to you.

- Keeping your journal will help you cope with the changes in your life.

- Attracting attention, sexual and social, may intimidate you.

- If diet boredom sets in, rediscover your enthusiasm by shaking things up or re-reading your diet book.

Chapter 6

Substances That Throw Up Roadblocks

In This Chapter

- Stalling in your diet has many reasons
- Kicking alcohol and tobacco
- Consuming chocolate and caffeine can be perilous
- Taking certain drugs may block loss
- Interacting for help

You may be following your diet to the letter. Balancing your nutrients, calculating points, counting carbs, figuring calories—all the mechanics of your plan—may be second nature to you now. But there might come a time when you just can't seem to lose any weight.

First on your to-do list when this happens: Start looking at the background noise in your diet. These items are things that may be so common that you don't think twice about taking them.

In this chapter, you'll find some of the substances that can throw a speed bump in front of your weight-loss rate. You'll find out how to counter their effects by using the interactive forms we've included to help you get a handle on what these substances do in your body. You'll also find out that some over-the-counter and prescription drugs can put the brakes on your diet. Finally, we will tell you why you have to watch out for those two ubiquitous drugs: caffeine and alcohol.

As always, however, you should never stop or change the dosage on a prescription drug without talking to your doctor first.

Drop That Lighter—Now

Every diet has different taboos, but there's at least one area where they all meet and agree: smoking. Studies have been cited for years on how smoking damages the lungs and can lead to various kinds of cancers. As if cancer weren't reason enough to quit, this habit can also play havoc with weight loss.

One word of advice: Don't try to begin a diet at the same time you are trying to quit smoking.

To do one of these activities well takes enormous self-discipline and desire; to do both of them at the same time may be taking on too much. Quitting smoking is extremely important, but you need to clear just one hurdle at a time.

> **Check This Out**
>
> About 4,000 chemicals are wafting around in that cigarette smoke, and 40 of them cause cancer.

> **Check This Out**
>
> Smokers are not as sensitive to insulin as nonsmokers, which means that if a smoker eats carbohydrates and his blood sugar spikes, it would take more insulin to bring his blood sugar level back to normal than it would for a nonsmoker.

Okay, you been told for decades what tobacco can do to your lungs, heart, blood vessels, and other organs, but what does smoking have to do with the way you digest food?

There are various theories. One is that the body reacts to lighting up a cigarette and inhaling the smoke the same way it would react to any sudden change: Among other actions, the body releases stress hormones and insulin. If you keep smoking, the body's organs seem to become less sensitive to insulin, so the body responds to that insensitivity by releasing even more insulin in an effort to overcome the insensitivity. The other end of this self-stoking cycle begins when you quit smoking. Quitting is another sudden change, so the body reacts as it would normally when faced with a sudden change or some other stress: It releases stress hormones and insulin.

The real question is: If insulin levels are high both when you start smoking and when you quit—why is it that you don't feel as hungry when you're smoking as you do just after you've quit?

That is the million-dollar question, and one that no one has a definitive answer for. Some scientists think that the nicotine in tobacco speeds up the metabolism enough so that it damps the cravings that raised insulin might ordinarily give you. When you quit smoking, there's no counterweight to the raised insulin levels, so you feel the full force of your cravings. Hence, the hunger and weight gain.

The bottom line is: Quit smoking. If you can't do it alone, join a support group. A little accountability—knowing you have to go to a meeting and confess your behavior—goes a long way toward making you think before you light up.

> **Check This Out**
>
> Within 12 hours of your last cigarette, your body is already starting to heal from the effects of nicotine.

In the same way that keeping a journal helps you diet, keeping a journal of your smoking may also help you break this habit. Seeing when, how much, and why you light up may help you think before you strike the match. If you think first, you may stick the cigarette back in the pack. And if you reconsider once, you can reconsider until you've kicked the habit.

> **Tips to Use**
>
> Skip the coffee—and anything else with caffeine in it. Withdrawing from tobacco's nicotine can make you jittery; you don't need caffeine compounding the side effect.

Check Here to Quit

Start the Smoking Checklist table by filling in the date. For instance, begin with the initial of the day of the week (M, Tu, W, Th, F, Sa, Su, for example) followed by the exact date (8-16 would represent Aug. 16, for instance). Under *Smoke #* write 1, 2, 3, and so on to represent whether this is your first, second, third, or more time lighting up. Under *Time*, list what time it was that you smoked. Under *What I Was Doing*, list your activity (answering the phone, starting the car, drinking, and so on) when you lit up.

If you keep this diary for at least a week, you'll be able to pick out your smoking patterns. For instance, if you only smoke when you answer the phone, recognize that as a habit you should break and do something such as have a glass of water in the hand that's not holding the phone. You'll do two things that way: You won't smoke, and you'll be drinking some of your diet's daily requirement of water. Under *To Break This Habit I Will* ..., list what you will do when the urge to smoke strikes you. This column doesn't have to be filled in every time you have a cigarette, but you should insert at least one goal a week here—and then put forward the effort to follow your own advice.

Smoking Checklist

Date	Smoke #	Time	What I Was Doing	To Break This Habit I Will ...

Give Alcohol the Big Chill

Many diets say alcohol drunk in moderation is probably good for you. The key word in this sentence, though, is *moderation*. By now, the term *French paradox* has permeated all levels of the drinking class. The French paradox refers to the fact that the French diet is much higher in saturated fat than an American diet, yet the French have fewer cancers and less death from heart disease. Many studies say this is because the French drink more wine than we do. However, this seeming contradiction between good living and low rates of heart disease is not a license to uncork your lunch. Rather, it is one piece of a very complex puzzle that you may want to incorporate into your diet.

Some diet authors encourage you to avoid alcohol because they feel your body will burn the alcohol instead of the fat. Even so, these authors acknowledge that there is some benefit to moderate or light drinking and say an occasional glass is fine, as long as you're not diabetic or can't control your drinking. Still other authors say that drinking impairs the liver's ability to detoxify your body, and alcohol should be avoided.

> **Check This Out**
>
> How much alcohol is *moderate*? An extensive study done by Harvard Medical School, along with other institutions, says that the greatest benefit to your heart and blood vessels occurs when people drink about one drink a day. Some data suggest that level should be slightly lower for women.

Obviously, if you have physical or addictive problems with alcohol, then eliminating it completely is probably the best course of action.

Consult your diet book to see what your plan calls for.

Caffeine: Different Person, Different Reaction

No drug saturates our society the way caffeine does. It's in candy; it's in soft drinks; it's in chocolate; it's in that early morning eye opener, coffee. It's a staple of restaurants and cafés. It's also a hotly debated stimulant.

Advice about it runs the gamut: One diet author says generally any fluid, including coffee and tea, counts toward the fluid you should take in each day, and so they're both fine. Another author says you should stop drinking caffeine in the beginning of your diet, but after you've been on the plan for a while, you can drink it again. Still another author says that drinking it is acceptable in the beginning of the diet, but you should aim to taper off and finally eliminate it altogether. Others say that you should see how your body reacts to caffeine and adjust accordingly.

> **Diet Alert**
>
> If you're sensitive to caffeine, be careful of over-the-counter drugs. This stimulant is often added to pain relievers, appetite suppressants, and cold medicines.

Dieters themselves report a range of effects from caffeine, from almost none at all to stalls in their weight loss.

If you drink high-octane coffee and have to peel yourself off of the ceiling, clutching a donut in each hand, you should seriously think about weaning yourself off of caffeine. If, however, caffeine doesn't make you jumpy, jittery, or start food cravings, you may be one of the lucky ones who can enjoy a cup of java and not be bothered by it. And, remember, you can always switch to decaffeinated drinks.

Think Twice About Chocolate

Some people swear that they are addicted to chocolate, and science bears them out to some extent. Sure, the fat, texture, smell, and sugar are the basis for some of the cravings, but there is evidence that it feeds a physical need, as well. According to some scientists, if you lack magnesium, or if you need to balance the brain chemicals involved in regulating mood and eating, having chocolate could be a form of self-medication.

In addition to being one of the most sensual of foods (has anyone ever given you gift-wrapped broccoli for Valentine's Day? We thought not ….), it is also one of the major foods that contain caffeine, and, as such, carries with it the potential drawbacks of the drug.

The following is a table that lays out exactly what level of caffeine some popular chocolate foods contain.

What's in Your Favorite Chocolate Foods?

Food	Portion Size	Caffeine (mg)
Baking chocolate, unsweetened	1 oz.	58
Brownies	1	1–3
Dark chocolate	1.45 oz. bar	30
Milk chocolate	1.55 oz. bar	11

Food	Portion Size	Caffeine (mg)
Semisweet chocolate chips	¼ cup	26–28
Cocoa-containing cereal	1 oz.	1
Chocolate chip cookies	1	1
Chocolate cupcake/ chocolate frosting	1	1–2
Fudge	1 piece	2–3
Ice cream/frozen yogurt	½ cup	2
Chocolate syrup, thin	1 TB.	3
Chocolate syrup, fudge-type	1 TB.	1

Even if you brush off the caffeine content of these chocolate foods, the other nutrients in them should give you pause for thought. For instance, that 17-gram piece of chocolate fudge with only about 2 or so milligrams of caffeine packs on 65 calories, 1 gram of fat, negligible protein, and nearly 14 grams of digestible carbohydrates.

Also, caffeine can have a diuretic effect. If you're on a diet that is naturally diuretic, such as a low-carb diet, this doubled effect may dehydrate you. If you're dehydrated, you'll likely be thirsty; the body sometimes confuses thirst with that of hunger. In other words, coffee may make you thirsty, but your body may think you're hungry and start craving food. Too many food cravings can lead to overeating, and overeating is why you had to start your diet in the first place.

> ### Check This Out
>
> Why is caffeine such a stumbling block? In the short term, it can make your cells less sensitive to insulin, triggering a cascade of body reactions. This results in far too much insulin being produced to normalize your blood sugar (according to a 2004 Harvard study).

> ### Check This Out
>
> Coffee showed up in Europe in 1615 thanks to some Venetian traders, an event that completed the great triumvirate of hot, caffeine-rich beverages. Hot chocolate had been on the scene since 1528 when the Spanish brought it back from the Americas, and tea had been in the marketplace since 1610.

Pluses and Minuses of Hormone Treatments

Women are commonly prescribed some kind of hormone replacement therapy if they're having extreme hot flashes or any of a range of problems before, during, or after menopause, or after the woman has had a hysterectomy or her ovaries removed. Birth control pills also have a certain amount of estrogen in them, which, in addition to the normally circulating hormones in her body, may make her retain more water and gain more weight than usual. But every woman is different. Not every older woman wants or needs hormone therapy for menopause; not every woman has a reaction to birth control pills.

Because women's hormones normally fluctuate, this variation can cause women to lose weight in fits and starts throughout the month.

Men don't get away from this issue unscathed. Men produce estrogen as well as testosterone.

The older a man is, the more likely it is that his testosterone levels will go down. When testosterone goes down, the estrogen effects are not as disguised. When estrogen is more of an active hormonal partner, losing weight or maintaining it may be harder.

A number of diet authors feel hormone therapies and even birth control pills upset a normal hormone balance and also affect the liver negatively. Hormone therapy may also slow weight loss, increase water retention, and spark cravings, some experts feel.

> **Check This Out**
>
> When a man is young, he makes enough testosterone that it dampens the effects of estrogen. This is why a normally healthy young man will have facial hair and not pronounced breasts.

> **CAUTION**
>
> **Diet Alert**
>
> Talk to your doctor before dropping or even changing the dosage of any medication you're taking. The reason you're on hormone therapy may far outweigh the need to lose weight rapidly. Above all, talk to your doctor and discuss with him or her the possibility of finding a compromise between your treatment and your diet plan.

High Blood Pressure Medications and Weight Loss

Being overweight is a major factor for high blood pressure, so getting thinner might make your blood pressure normal—but don't bet on it. Weight loss doesn't automatically lead to normal blood pressure, but the good news is that it can and has for many people.

It helps to know that the very medication that may be saving your life may also be affecting your weight loss to some degree. Among the side effects for various kinds of high blood pressure medicines are bloating, constipation, low potassium, and other symptoms. Also, if you're on a low-carb diet, you need to be aware that high blood pressure medicine may make your insulin levels rise.

Regardless of the type of diet you're on, if you have stopped losing weight, there could be many reasons for it, not just this medication.

As you lose weight, you will want to check with your doctor frequently. If your weight goes down enough, your blood pressure may also go down, and your doctor might want to change your medication. But never, ever change it on your own.

> **CAUTION**
>
> **Diet Alert** _____
>
> It is crucial to talk to your doctor before changing your dose or stopping it altogether. Never experiment on your own with your high blood pressure medication; you may be setting yourself up for a stroke or heart attack.

The Debate on Cholesterol-Reducing Drugs

The debate here among some diet authors is whether high cholesterol levels in your bloodstream really mean that you'll die sooner. Some say studies are inconclusive and don't show that high cholesterol levels contribute to an early death. Other experts say high levels of cholesterol in your bloodstream are linked to heart disease. All agree, however, that watching what you eat—and eating less—will very likely reduce the most harmful kinds of cholesterol.

About 80 percent of your cholesterol is made by your own liver and does not come from your diet. So, basically, when you're taking a cholesterol-reducing drug, you're trying to counter your body's natural tendency to produce a lot of this waxy compound that helps strengthen cells and is needed to produce various hormones.

Because the liver is so involved both in making cholesterol and processing blood sugar and fat, drugs that affect this organ's function are viewed warily by many diet experts.

> **CAUTION**
>
> **Diet Alert** _____
>
> Even though your diet book may show you case histories that sound just like you, _they are not you_. Every person can have a different reaction to a specific diet. Monitor your own health carefully, and never, ever mistake the general observations in any diet book for specific medical advice aimed at you personally.

If you are taking a cholesterol-lowering drug, talk to your doctor before changing your dose or stopping the drug.

The Danger in Corticosteroids

Corticosteroids are drugs that counter inflammation, particularly in chronic diseases such as rheumatoid arthritis and asthma. They even help minor ailments such as itching and rashes. They can be a miracle of pain relief for some people, but, as with everything, the good these drugs do comes with a price. Among the possible side effects are weight gain and water retention, not to mention bone loss, muscle wasting, mood swings, and more.

The last two side effects are obviously at odds with your diet, but, even if your weight loss is slowed, you should never experiment with the dosage on these drugs. If you are on any corticosteroid, never, ever stop it without talking to your doctor first.

Even if you've only taken a corticosteroid for a couple of weeks, suddenly eliminating it may cause life-threatening adrenal failure. Your adrenal glands sit on top of your kidneys, and they are the glands that produce a range of hormones that, among other functions, respond to stress by raising blood pressure, increasing heart rate, and elevating blood sugar. In fact, if you take any corticosteroid long term, your adrenal glands may not respond properly for up to a year after you've stopped taking the drug. This means that you may have trouble recovering from surgery, infection, or some other stress.

What's That Mean?

Anabolic steroids are man-made chemicals that mimic the effects of male sex hormones. Bodybuilders and athletes many times use them to increase muscle mass. Side effects can include sterility, heart attack, and serious liver problems, among other effects.

Corticosteroids, by the way, should not be confused with *anabolic steroids*, which have a degree of infamy attached to them. Anabolic steroids can pump up your muscles much like testosterone does and have been used illegally by athletes and others who want more mass.

Side Effects of Antidepressants

Some experts say high levels of insulin over the long term can pave the way for depression and other illnesses. A careful diet can sharpen the interaction of chemical messengers in the brain and lift depression, says another expert. Still another expert believes that very low levels of insulin can lead to depression because the pancreatic hormone is the key in triggering the release of a mood-enhancing, brain-messenger chemical called *serotonin*. He further believes that too little serotonin can lead to depression.

Dozens of drugs on the market treat depression, and there is no one-size-fits-all prescription. Many of these drugs have side effects that range from dry mouth and sleepiness to dizziness. They can also have weight gain as a side effect, and this is why your doctor's choice of antidepressant may have an effect on your diet.

If you think your antidepressant is slowing your weight loss, see your doctor and talk over the options. Many times, there is an alternate drug your doctor can give you that may not have the same side effects. Sometimes, however, your doctor may want to keep you on your current antidepressant. Listen to your doctor.

As with any prescribed medication, don't stop it or change the dosage on your own.

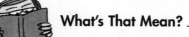

What's That Mean?

Serotonin is a brain chemical that is key in regulating mood, appetite, sleep, body temperature, blood pressure, heartbeat, and other functions.

Diet Alert

Taking care of some medical conditions comes first; losing weight comes second. Besides, there is no hard-and-fast timetable for your weight loss; if you do it more slowly than your neighbor—so what?

The Trouble with Herbals and Over-the-Counter Drugs

Just because something grows in your yard, or you buy it at the health food store, or you pick it up at the checkout counter at the corner drugstore, don't assume these plants, herbs, and over-the-counter drugs are harmless.

Many times substances such as antacids and stool softeners can raise your insulin levels. When your insulin levels are raised, you tend to crave carbohydrates. When you crave carbohydrates, you may go on an eating binge, and when that happens, you gain weight.

Ephedrine is probably the most controversial of the substances that dieters mention taking. However, not one diet we studied suggests taking this herbal, and we found no reliable expert who endorsed this substance. Using this stimulant, however, is much discussed on bulletin boards and chat rooms, with some dieters attesting to its virtues and others cautioning against side effects that can be severe, and even fatal.

It doesn't matter what the underground word is on this herbal, however. The FDA, as of April 2004, banned the sale of any dietary supplement containing ephedrine alkaloids (ephedra). This substance in recent years has been linked to a number of deaths, including that of a 23-year-old prospective pitcher for the Baltimore Orioles in 2003. He had taken three ephedra pills on an empty stomach, said the coroner, and, combined with other health issues and a hot day, ended up dying. Dozens more deaths have been linked to this herbal.

What's That Mean?

Ephedrine is the main active ingredient in ephedra (also called Ma huang), and is a naturally occurring substance that comes from plants. Ephedra is a stimulant that acts like adrenaline and may have dangerous effects on the heart and blood pressure.

So why are we bringing ephedra up if it's banned? There's a loophole in the ruling. The FDA's ban doesn't generally apply to items such as herbal teas that are regulated as conventional foods. The ban also doesn't apply to traditional Chinese herbal remedies.

The best advice we can offer: Don't take any substance that contains ephedrine alkaloids.

Cough Drops and Chewing Gum

Cough drops, cough syrups, and chewing gum may seem innocuous enough, but these are items where it pays to read the nutritional label information.

For instance, many cough drops and syrups contain sugar in one form or another, and added sugar is not desirable in any diet. If you find out this is the case with the brand you're fond of, try looking for it in a sugar-free version.

Chewing gum doesn't even seem like a food. You just chew and chew and chew and never actually eat it, so why do you have to be careful of it?

Check This Out

Ancient Greeks chewed gum made from the resin of the mastic tree; ancient Mayans made it from the sap (chicle) of the sapodilla tree; and Native Americans used sap from spruce trees as gum.

Actually, the reaction among diet experts on chewing gum runs the gamut from no reaction at all, regarding it as a good substitute for a snack, or completely eliminating it from your food list.

Why do some diet authors think chewing gum is so bad? They say that the chewing action and the sweet taste fools your body into thinking it's about to digest something. The body gears up by increasing insulin, and then, because little to no energy is taken in, the insulin levels stay high. When insulin levels are high, and there is no food in the off-ing, your cravings increase. Increased cravings usually mean more eating. More eating means more weight gain. The diet plans that want you to cross chewing gum off of your list are aiming to short circuit this parade of events.

This is the last page of your guide, but it is the jumping off place where the work really begins. Remember all the advice and cautions we've given you, and use them to go forward into your new lifestyle. Keep your daily food diaries meticulously; the more detailed you make them, the more they will help you. Also, use the nutritional food table we've provided. It doesn't matter if you're counting calories, counting car-bohydrates, counting fat, or simply following portion sizes, the nutritional guide will give you the information you need to keep to your plan and keep losing weight. Along with your growing self-confidence and self-discipline, the tools in this book will be your biggest assets in your weight-loss plan. And remember: Never, ever give up!

The Least You Need to Know

- ◆ The most common things you eat, drink, or take as drugs may be slowing your weight loss.

- ◆ No doctor-prescribed drug or its dosage should ever be changed unless your doctor says it's all right.

- ◆ Try to quit smoking before you start your diet; doing two discipline-heavy things at the same time may sabotage both.

- ◆ Limit—or eliminate—alcohol in your diet.

- ◆ Never give up!

My Food Journal

Your food journal is the heart of your diet. And, yes, we know, the record-keeping portion of your diet is not the part that makes your smile brighter and your step lighter. But, just consider this: When you stall or plateau, you'll be able to see, 9 times out of 10, exactly where you went wrong and be able to lift yourself off of your stall or plateau with a minimum of hair tearing.

Also, there's the feel-good aspect about keeping a food and exercise journal. In the coming months, you'll be able to look back across the expanse of your own personal dieting landscape and see how far you've come. The chocolate cookies and dinner rolls have tapered off into poached salmon and salads, and you've seen the pounds roll off and your "fat" clothes hang loosely. Nothing feels better. But that euphoria is hard-won, and keeping a food journal is strongly urged by nearly every diet expert.

We've provided enough daily forms for you to get you started, but you'll probably need more as time goes on. Please, help yourself. Feel free to make as many copies of the basic form as you need. Many people, in fact, find it helpful to compile their food journals in a separate notebook. Each day's journal begins by filling in the day's date—and don't forget to include the year, at least in the beginning. It's surprising how time flies, and you want to be certain when you've reached a milestone. Next, write your weight in the provided space. Some diets want you to weigh yourself every day, some occasionally, and some not at all. Follow your own diet plan.

The weather may seem irrelevant, but it's amazing to see how a sunny day may correlate with an upbeat mood, and a week of dank, chilly, rainy days may put you in a funk. Keeping track of this tidbit may help you analyze when mood swings are not totally related to hormone or other intrinsic body activities.

Below this information are two sets of boxes. The first set on the left is labeled *Water*. As you drink the glasses of water required by your diet, put a check mark in the boxes. It's an easy way to see if you've drunk enough every day. Keeping track will also help you if you have side effects such as constipation. Many times these side effects are the result of simply not drinking enough water.

To the right of *Water* are check boxes for your vitamin and other supplements. Nearly all diet experts encourage some form of added nutrients. If you take a daily multivitamin, put a check in the box next to the label, *I took my vitamin*. If you're supplementing in any other way, check the box labeled *Other supplements*. You'll never again hold a bottle in one hand while asking the face in the bathroom mirror whether you've already taken your pills.

Below these boxes is the heart of the form: your food diary. Fill in the foods you eat for each meal and at each snack time. On the right side in this area are columns headed with the words *Pro*, *Fat*, *Carb*, *Pts or Cal*. If you're on a low-carb diet, you'll pay more attention to the first three columns where you will write in the amounts of protein, fat, and carbohydrates each food has. Other diets require keeping track of points, exchanges, or calories. Put that number in the last column. Many diets want each meal to be balanced for whatever nutrients they require, which is why the subtotal line is there. At the end of the day, you can total what you've had and see readily if you've kept to your diet. Just a reminder for low-carb dieters: The carbohydrate count is what's left after you subtract the dietary fiber.

Next is the section to help you reach your goals on exercise. Take your heart rate before you start exercising, which is your resting heart rate, and write it down. Then, take your heart rate again when you've reached maximum effort and write that down; this will tell you if you're reaching your target heart rate—the rate your heart should pump to get the most benefit from the exercise. Don't forget to write down your goals. These can be your long-term goals or goals you have for the next day. Seeing your target written out will help you mentally prepare for the next push.

Below your goals, check the exercise boxes that apply to you. Are you doing light, medium, or heavy exercising? How long are you doing it for? Don't forget to write down exactly what the exercise was (walking, running, tennis, and so on).

Below the exercise area, you'll see two areas that will help you see where you are mentally. Put a check in the boxes that reflect most closely the way you feel. Your state of mind is important because that will tell you if something is bothering you. You can check more than one box here, say, if you're feeling both angry and frustrated. If you don't feel like any of these choices, you can either skip this area or cross out a choice and write in your own. The important thing here is to be frank about your feelings.

Your sleep log is important because tiredness is one of the major triggers people cite for going off of their diets. There will always be restless nights, but if not sleeping becomes a pattern, you will want to know about this. If this pattern begins to disrupt your waking life, you will want to speak to your doctor and show him or her your journals.

The blank space at the bottom of the form is both to record your comments and thoughts and also to prime you to try to do better the next day. You might be surprised at how much these comments will mean to you months from now when you need a little inspiration. These comments are a way of talking to the person you will become and remembering who you were after you've reached your goal.

Sample

Date 04/01/05	My Weight 165		Weather 65 deg.

Water ☐ ☐ ☐ ☐   I took my vitamin   ☑
☑ ☑ ☑ ☐   Other supplements   ☐

Food Diary

Breakfast	Pro	Fat	Carb	Pts or Cal
2 poached eggs	12	10	2	150
3 slices bacon	6	9	0	109
Coffee	0	0	1	4
	—	—	—	—
	—	—	—	—
Subtotal	18	19	3	263

Lunch	Pro	Fat	Carb	Pts or Cal
Sm. chicken breast, roasted	54	6	0	284
Broccoli, 1 cup	3	0	2.4	25
Herb tea	0	0	0	2
	—	—	—	—
	—	—	—	—
Subtotal	57	6	2.4	311

Dinner	Pro	Fat	Carb	Pts or Cal
Broiled pork, 3 oz.	24	11	0	204
Barbecue sauce, 1 tsp.	0	0	1.8	12
Lettuce, 1 cup	1	0	0.2	7
Bleu cheese dressing, 1 tsp.	1	8	1	77
Subtotal	26	19	3	300

Snacks	Pro	Fat	Carb	Pts or Cal
Macadamia nuts, $\frac{1}{2}$ cup	5	51	3.1	480
Whole orange	1	0	12	62
Day's Total	119	113	23.5	1,416

Date _04/01/05_   **My Weight** _165_   **Weather** _65 deg._

Heart rate:
Resting: _____   Max: _____

My goals:
Weight: _____   Heart rate (max): _____

My mood is
❏ Happy   ❏ Ordinary   ❏ Sad

My current state of mind is (check all that apply)
❏ Angry ❏ Frustrated ❏ Determined ❏ Anxious ❏ Not feeling well ❏ Tired
☑ Optimistic ☑ Stressed ❏ Other

I slept
❏ Soundly ☑ Average ❏ Below average ❏ Not at all

Exercise was
❏ Light   ❏ Less than 10 min.
❏ Medium   ☑ 10–30 min.
❏ Intense   ❏ 30–60 min.

I need to pay more attention to *upping my carb count and lowering my fat.*
Also, I'm behind at work, and it's stressing me out. Tomorrow I'll clear my
desk. Someone complimented me on how thin I look—that felt terrific! Drink
more water!

My Food Journal

Date _____   My Weight _____   Weather _____

Water ☐☐☐☐   I took my vitamin   ☐
      ☐☐☐☐   Other supplements   ☐

Food Diary

Breakfast	Pro	Fat	Carb	Pts or Cal
_____	—	—	—	—
_____	—	—	—	—
_____	—	—	—	—
_____	—	—	—	—
_____	—	—	—	—
Subtotal	—	—	—	—

Lunch	Pro	Fat	Carb	Pts or Cal
_____	—	—	—	—
_____	—	—	—	—
_____	—	—	—	—
_____	—	—	—	—
_____	—	—	—	—
Subtotal	—	—	—	—

Dinner	Pro	Fat	Carb	Pts or Cal
_____	—	—	—	—
_____	—	—	—	—
_____	—	—	—	—
_____	—	—	—	—
Subtotal	—	—	—	—

Snacks	Pro	Fat	Carb	Pts or Cal
_____	—	—	—	—
_____	—	—	—	—
	—	—	—	—
Day's Total	—	—	—	—

Date _____   **My Weight** _____   **Weather** _____

Heart rate:
Resting: _____   Max: _____

My goals:
Weight: _____   Heart rate (max) _____

My mood is
❑ Happy   ❑ Ordinary   ❑ Sad

My current state of mind is (check all that apply)
❑ Angry ❑ Frustrated ❑ Determined ❑ Anxious ❑ Not feeling well ❑ Tired
❑ Optimistic ❑ Stressed ❑ Other

I slept
❑ Soundly ❑ Average ❑ Below average ❑ Not at all

Exercise was
❑ Light   ❑ Less than 10 min.
❑ Medium   ❑ 10–30 min.
❑ Intense   ❑ 30–60 min.

I need to pay more attention to _____

_____

_____

_____

_____

My Food Journal

Date _____   My Weight _____   Weather _____

Water ☐☐☐☐   I took my vitamin   ☐
      ☐☐☐☐   Other supplements   ☐

Food Diary

Breakfast	Pro	Fat	Carb	Pts or Cal
_____	—	—	—	—
_____	—	—	—	—
_____	—	—	—	—
_____	—	—	—	—
_____	—	—	—	—
Subtotal	—	—	—	—

Lunch	Pro	Fat	Carb	Pts or Cal
_____	—	—	—	—
_____	—	—	—	—
_____	—	—	—	—
_____	—	—	—	—
_____	—	—	—	—
Subtotal	—	—	—	—

Dinner	Pro	Fat	Carb	Pts or Cal
_____	—	—	—	—
_____	—	—	—	—
_____	—	—	—	—
_____	—	—	—	—
_____	—	—	—	—
Subtotal	—	—	—	—

Snacks	Pro	Fat	Carb	Pts or Cal
_____	—	—	—	—
_____	—	—	—	—
_____	—	—	—	—
Day's Total	—	—	—	—

Date _____   **My Weight** _____   **Weather** _____

Heart rate:
Resting: ____   Max: ____

My goals:
Weight: ____   Heart rate (max) ____

My mood is
❏ Happy   ❏ Ordinary   ❏ Sad

My current state of mind is (check all that apply)
❏ Angry ❏ Frustrated ❏ Determined ❏ Anxious ❏ Not feeling well ❏ Tired
❏ Optimistic ❏ Stressed ❏ Other

I slept
❏ Soundly ❏ Average ❏ Below average ❏ Not at all

Exercise was
❏ Light   ❏ Less than 10 min.
❏ Medium   ❏ 10–30 min.
❏ Intense   ❏ 30–60 min.

I need to pay more attention to _____

_____

_____

_____

_____

My Food Journal

Date _____ My Weight _____ Weather _____

Water ☐☐☐☐
☐☐☐☐

I took my vitamin ☐
Other supplements ☐

Food Diary

Breakfast	Pro	Fat	Carb	Pts or Cal
_____	—	—	—	—
_____	—	—	—	—
_____	—	—	—	—
_____	—	—	—	—
_____	—	—	—	—
Subtotal	—	—	—	—

Lunch	Pro	Fat	Carb	Pts or Cal
_____	—	—	—	—
_____	—	—	—	—
_____	—	—	—	—
_____	—	—	—	—
_____	—	—	—	—
Subtotal	—	—	—	—

Dinner	Pro	Fat	Carb	Pts or Cal
_____	—	—	—	—
_____	—	—	—	—
_____	—	—	—	—
_____	—	—	—	—
_____	—	—	—	—
Subtotal	—	—	—	—

Snacks	Pro	Fat	Carb	Pts or Cal
_____	—	—	—	—
_____	—	—	—	—
_____	—	—	—	—
Day's Total	—	—	—	—

Date _____   **My Weight** _____   **Weather** _____

Heart rate:
Resting: ____   Max: ____

My goals:
Weight: ____   Heart rate (max) ____

My mood is
❏ Happy   ❏ Ordinary   ❏ Sad

My current state of mind is (check all that apply)
❏ Angry ❏ Frustrated ❏ Determined ❏ Anxious ❏ Not feeling well ❏ Tired
❏ Optimistic ❏ Stressed ❏ Other

I slept
❏ Soundly ❏ Average ❏ Below average ❏ Not at all

Exercise was
❏ Light   ❏ Less than 10 min.
❏ Medium   ❏ 10–30 min.
❏ Intense   ❏ 30–60 min.

I need to pay more attention to _____

_____

_____

_____

_____

My Food Journal

Date _____   My Weight _____   Weather _____

Water   ☐ ☐ ☐ ☐   I took my vitamin   ☐
          ☐ ☐ ☐ ☐   Other supplements   ☐

Food Diary

Breakfast	Pro	Fat	Carb	Pts or Cal
_____	—	—	—	—
_____	—	—	—	—
_____	—	—	—	—
_____	—	—	—	—
_____	—	—	—	—
Subtotal	—	—	—	—

Lunch	Pro	Fat	Carb	Pts or Cal
_____	—	—	—	—
_____	—	—	—	—
_____	—	—	—	—
_____	—	—	—	—
_____	—	—	—	—
Subtotal	—	—	—	—

Dinner	Pro	Fat	Carb	Pts or Cal
_____	—	—	—	—
_____	—	—	—	—
_____	—	—	—	—
_____	—	—	—	—
Subtotal	—	—	—	—

Snacks	Pro	Fat	Carb	Pts or Cal
_____	—	—	—	—
_____	—	—	—	—
_____	—	—	—	—
Day's Total	—	—	—	—

Date _____   **My Weight** _____   **Weather** _____

Heart rate:
Resting: ____   Max: ____

My goals:
Weight: ____   Heart rate (max) ____

My mood is
❏ Happy   ❏ Ordinary   ❏ Sad

My current state of mind is (check all that apply)
❏ Angry ❏ Frustrated ❏ Determined ❏ Anxious ❏ Not feeling well ❏ Tired
❏ Optimistic ❏ Stressed ❏ Other

I slept
❏ Soundly   ❏ Average   ❏ Below average   ❏ Not at all

Exercise was
❏ Light   ❏ Less than 10 min.
❏ Medium   ❏ 10–30 min.
❏ Intense   ❏ 30–60 min.

I need to pay more attention to _____

_____

_____

_____

_____

My Food Journal

Date _____   My Weight _____   Weather _____

Water ☐☐☐☐   I took my vitamin   ☐
      ☐☐☐☐   Other supplements   ☐

Food Diary

Breakfast	Pro	Fat	Carb	Pts or Cal
_____	——	——	——	——
_____	——	——	——	——
_____	——	——	——	——
_____	——	——	——	——
_____	——	——	——	——
Subtotal	——	——	——	——

Lunch	Pro	Fat	Carb	Pts or Cal
_____	——	——	——	——
_____	——	——	——	——
_____	——	——	——	——
_____	——	——	——	——
_____	——	——	——	——
Subtotal	——	——	——	——

Dinner	Pro	Fat	Carb	Pts or Cal
_____	——	——	——	——
_____	——	——	——	——
_____	——	——	——	——
_____	——	——	——	——
_____	——	——	——	——
Subtotal	——	——	——	——

Snacks	Pro	Fat	Carb	Pts or Cal
_____	——	——	——	——
_____	——	——	——	——
Day's Total	——	——	——	——

Date _____   **My Weight** _____   **Weather** _____

Heart rate:
Resting: _____   Max: _____

My goals:
Weight: _____   Heart rate (max) _____

My mood is
❏ Happy   ❏ Ordinary   ❏ Sad

My current state of mind is (check all that apply)
❏ Angry ❏ Frustrated ❏ Determined ❏ Anxious ❏ Not feeling well ❏ Tired
❏ Optimistic ❏ Stressed ❏ Other

I slept
❏ Soundly   ❏ Average   ❏ Below average   ❏ Not at all

Exercise was
❏ Light   ❏ Less than 10 min.
❏ Medium   ❏ 10–30 min.
❏ Intense   ❏ 30–60 min.

I need to pay more attention to _____

_____

_____

_____

_____

My Food Journal

Date _____   **My Weight** _____   **Weather** _____

Water ❏ ❏ ❏ ❏   I took my vitamin   ❏
       ❏ ❏ ❏ ❏   Other supplements   ❏

Food Diary

Breakfast	Pro	Fat	Carb	Pts or Cal
_____	—	—	—	—
_____	—	—	—	—
_____	—	—	—	—
_____	—	—	—	—
_____	—	—	—	—
Subtotal	—	—	—	—

Lunch	Pro	Fat	Carb	Pts or Cal
_____	—	—	—	—
_____	—	—	—	—
_____	—	—	—	—
_____	—	—	—	—
_____	—	—	—	—
Subtotal	—	—	—	—

Dinner	Pro	Fat	Carb	Pts or Cal
_____	—	—	—	—
_____	—	—	—	—
_____	—	—	—	—
_____	—	—	—	—
_____	—	—	—	—
Subtotal	—	—	—	—

Snacks	Pro	Fat	Carb	Pts or Cal
_____	—	—	—	—
_____	—	—	—	—
_____	—	—	—	—
Day's Total	—	—	—	—

Date _____   **My Weight** _____   **Weather** _____

Heart rate:
Resting: ____   Max: ____

My goals:
Weight: ____   Heart rate (max) ____

My mood is
❏ Happy   ❏ Ordinary   ❏ Sad

My current state of mind is (check all that apply)
❏ Angry ❏ Frustrated ❏ Determined ❏ Anxious ❏ Not feeling well ❏ Tired
❏ Optimistic ❏ Stressed ❏ Other

I slept
❏ Soundly   ❏ Average   ❏ Below average   ❏ Not at all

Exercise was
❏ Light   ❏ Less than 10 min.
❏ Medium   ❏ 10–30 min.
❏ Intense   ❏ 30–60 min.

I need to pay more attention to _____

_____

_____

_____

_____

My Food Journal

Date _____   My Weight _____   Weather _____

Water ☐☐☐☐   I took my vitamin   ☐
      ☐☐☐☐   Other supplements   ☐

Food Diary

Breakfast	Pro	Fat	Carb	Pts or Cal
_____	__	__	__	__
_____	__	__	__	__
_____	__	__	__	__
_____	__	__	__	__
Subtotal	__	__	__	__

Lunch	Pro	Fat	Carb	Pts or Cal
_____	__	__	__	__
_____	__	__	__	__
_____	__	__	__	__
_____	__	__	__	__
Subtotal	__	__	__	__

Dinner	Pro	Fat	Carb	Pts or Cal
_____	__	__	__	__
_____	__	__	__	__
_____	__	__	__	__
_____	__	__	__	__
Subtotal	__	__	__	__

Snacks	Pro	Fat	Carb	Pts or Cal
_____	__	__	__	__
_____	__	__	__	__
Day's Total	__	__	__	__

Date _____   **My Weight** _____   **Weather** _____

Heart rate:
Resting: _____   Max: _____

My goals:
Weight: _____   Heart rate (max) _____

My mood is
❏ Happy   ❏ Ordinary   ❏ Sad

My current state of mind is (check all that apply)
❏ Angry ❏ Frustrated ❏ Determined ❏ Anxious ❏ Not feeling well ❏ Tired
❏ Optimistic ❏ Stressed ❏ Other

I slept
❏ Soundly ❏ Average ❏ Below average ❏ Not at all

Exercise was
❏ Light   ❏ Less than 10 min.
❏ Medium   ❏ 10–30 min.
❏ Intense   ❏ 30–60 min.

I need to pay more attention to _____

_____

_____

_____

_____

My Food Journal

Date _____   My Weight _____   Weather _____

Water ☐☐☐☐   I took my vitamin   ☐
      ☐☐☐☐   Other supplements   ☐

Food Diary

Breakfast	Pro	Fat	Carb	Pts or Cal
_____	—	—	—	—
_____	—	—	—	—
_____	—	—	—	—
_____	—	—	—	—
_____	—	—	—	—
Subtotal	—	—	—	—

Lunch	Pro	Fat	Carb	Pts or Cal
_____	—	—	—	—
_____	—	—	—	—
_____	—	—	—	—
_____	—	—	—	—
_____	—	—	—	—
Subtotal	—	—	—	—

Dinner	Pro	Fat	Carb	Pts or Cal
_____	—	—	—	—
_____	—	—	—	—
_____	—	—	—	—
_____	—	—	—	—
_____	—	—	—	—
Subtotal	—	—	—	—

Snacks	Pro	Fat	Carb	Pts or Cal
_____	—	—	—	—
_____	—	—	—	—
_____	—	—	—	—
Day's Total	—	—	—	—

Date _____ **My Weight** _____ **Weather** _____

Heart rate:
Resting: ____   Max: ____

My goals:
Weight: ____   Heart rate (max) ____

My mood is
❑ Happy   ❑ Ordinary   ❑ Sad

My current state of mind is (check all that apply)
❑ Angry ❑ Frustrated ❑ Determined ❑ Anxious ❑ Not feeling well ❑ Tired
❑ Optimistic ❑ Stressed ❑ Other

I slept
❑ Soundly   ❑ Average   ❑ Below average   ❑ Not at all

Exercise was
❑ Light   ❑ Less than 10 min.
❑ Medium   ❑ 10–30 min.
❑ Intense   ❑ 30–60 min.

I need to pay more attention to _____

_____

_____

_____

My Food Journal

Date _____   My Weight _____   Weather _____

Water ☐☐☐☐   I took my vitamin   ☐
☐☐☐☐   Other supplements   ☐

Food Diary

Breakfast	Pro	Fat	Carb	Pts or Cal
_____	—	—	—	—
_____	—	—	—	—
_____	—	—	—	—
_____	—	—	—	—
_____	—	—	—	—
Subtotal	—	—	—	—

Lunch	Pro	Fat	Carb	Pts or Cal
_____	—	—	—	—
_____	—	—	—	—
_____	—	—	—	—
_____	—	—	—	—
Subtotal	—	—	—	—

Dinner	Pro	Fat	Carb	Pts or Cal
_____	—	—	—	—
_____	—	—	—	—
_____	—	—	—	—
_____	—	—	—	—
Subtotal	—	—	—	—

Snacks	Pro	Fat	Carb	Pts or Cal
_____	—	—	—	—
_____	—	—	—	—
_____	—	—	—	—
Day's Total	—	—	—	—

Date _____ **My Weight** _____ **Weather** _____

Heart rate:
Resting: _____ Max: _____

My goals:
Weight: _____ Heart rate (max) _____

My mood is
❏ Happy ❏ Ordinary ❏ Sad

My current state of mind is (check all that apply)
❏ Angry ❏ Frustrated ❏ Determined ❏ Anxious ❏ Not feeling well ❏ Tired
❏ Optimistic ❏ Stressed ❏ Other

I slept
❏ Soundly ❏ Average ❏ Below average ❏ Not at all

Exercise was
❏ Light ❏ Less than 10 min.
❏ Medium ❏ 10–30 min.
❏ Intense ❏ 30–60 min.

I need to pay more attention to _____

_____

_____

_____

_____

My Food Journal

Date _____   **My Weight** _____   **Weather** _____

Water ❑ ❑ ❑ ❑   I took my vitamin   ❑
      ❑ ❑ ❑ ❑   Other supplements   ❑

Food Diary

Breakfast	Pro	Fat	Carb	Pts or Cal
_____	—	—	—	—
_____	—	—	—	—
_____	—	—	—	—
_____	—	—	—	—
_____	—	—	—	
Subtotal	—	—	—	—

Lunch	Pro	Fat	Carb	Pts or Cal
_____	—	—	—	—
_____	—	—	—	—
_____	—	—	—	—
_____	—	—	—	—
Subtotal	—	—	—	—

Dinner	Pro	Fat	Carb	Pts or Cal
_____	—	—	—	—
_____	—	—	—	—
_____	—	—	—	—
_____	—	—	—	—
Subtotal	—	—	—	—

Snacks	Pro	Fat	Carb	Pts or Cal
_____	—	—	—	—
_____	—	—	—	—
Day's Total	—	—	—	—

Date _____   **My Weight** _____   **Weather** _____

Heart rate:
Resting: _____   Max: _____

My goals:
Weight: _____   Heart rate (max) _____

My mood is
❑ Happy   ❑ Ordinary   ❑ Sad

My current state of mind is (check all that apply)
❑ Angry ❑ Frustrated ❑ Determined ❑ Anxious ❑ Not feeling well ❑ Tired
❑ Optimistic ❑ Stressed ❑ Other

I slept
❑ Soundly ❑ Average ❑ Below average ❑ Not at all

Exercise was
❑ Light   ❑ Less than 10 min.
❑ Medium   ❑ 10–30 min.
❑ Intense   ❑ 30–60 min.

I need to pay more attention to _____

_____

_____

_____

_____

My Food Journal

Date _____   My Weight _____   Weather _____

Water ☐ ☐ ☐ ☐   I took my vitamin   ☐
       ☐ ☐ ☐ ☐   Other supplements   ☐

Food Diary

Breakfast	Pro	Fat	Carb	Pts or Cal
_____	—	—	—	—
_____	—	—	—	—
_____	—	—	—	—
_____	—	—	—	—
_____	—	—	—	—
Subtotal	—	—	—	—

Lunch	Pro	Fat	Carb	Pts or Cal
_____	—	—	—	—
_____	—	—	—	—
_____	—	—	—	—
_____	—	—	—	—
_____	—	—	—	—
Subtotal	—	—	—	—

Dinner	Pro	Fat	Carb	Pts or Cal
_____	—	—	—	—
_____	—	—	—	—
_____	—	—	—	—
_____	—	—	—	—
_____	—	—	—	—
Subtotal	—	—	—	—

Snacks	Pro	Fat	Carb	Pts or Cal
_____	—	—	—	—
_____	—	—	—	—
Day's Total	—	—	—	—

Date _____ **My Weight** _____ **Weather** _____

Heart rate:
Resting: ____ Max: ____

My goals:
Weight: ____ Heart rate (max) ____

My mood is
❑ Happy ❑ Ordinary ❑ Sad

My current state of mind is (check all that apply)
❑ Angry ❑ Frustrated ❑ Determined ❑ Anxious ❑ Not feeling well ❑ Tired
❑ Optimistic ❑ Stressed ❑ Other

I slept
❑ Soundly ❑ Average ❑ Below average ❑ Not at all

Exercise was
❑ Light   ❑ Less than 10 min.
❑ Medium   ❑ 10–30 min.
❑ Intense   ❑ 30–60 min.

I need to pay more attention to _____

_____

_____

_____

_____

My Food Journal

Date _____   My Weight _____   Weather _____

Water ☐☐☐☐   I took my vitamin   ☐
      ☐☐☐☐   Other supplements   ☐

Food Diary

Breakfast	Pro	Fat	Carb	Pts or Cal
_____	—	—	—	—
_____	—	—	—	—
_____	—	—	—	—
_____	—	—	—	—
_____	—	—	—	—
Subtotal	—	—	—	—

Lunch	Pro	Fat	Carb	Pts or Cal
_____	—	—	—	—
_____	—	—	—	—
_____	—	—	—	—
_____	—	—	—	—
_____	—	—	—	—
Subtotal	—	—	—	—

Dinner	Pro	Fat	Carb	Pts or Cal
_____	—	—	—	—
_____	—	—	—	—
_____	—	—	—	—
_____	—	—	—	—
Subtotal	—	—	—	—

Snacks	Pro	Fat	Carb	Pts or Cal
_____	—	—	—	—
_____	—	—	—	—
_____	—	—	—	—
Day's Total	—	—	—	—

Date _____   **My Weight** _____   **Weather** _____

Heart rate:
Resting: ____   Max: ____

My goals:
Weight: ____   Heart rate (max) ____

My mood is
❏ Happy   ❏ Ordinary   ❏ Sad

My current state of mind is (check all that apply)
❏ Angry ❏ Frustrated ❏ Determined ❏ Anxious ❏ Not feeling well ❏ Tired
❏ Optimistic ❏ Stressed ❏ Other

I slept
❏ Soundly   ❏ Average   ❏ Below average   ❏ Not at all

Exercise was
❏ Light   ❏ Less than 10 min.
❏ Medium   ❏ 10–30 min.
❏ Intense   ❏ 30–60 min.

I need to pay more attention to _____

_____

_____

_____

_____

My Food Journal

Date _____   **My Weight** _____   **Weather** _____

Water ☐ ☐ ☐ ☐   I took my vitamin   ☐
       ☐ ☐ ☐ ☐   Other supplements   ☐

Food Diary

Breakfast	Pro	Fat	Carb	Pts or Cal
_____	—	—	—	—
_____	—	—	—	—
_____	—	—	—	—
_____	—	—	—	—
_____	—	—	—	—
Subtotal	—	—	—	—

Lunch	Pro	Fat	Carb	Pts or Cal
_____	—	—	—	—
_____	—	—	—	—
_____	—	—	—	—
_____	—	—	—	—
Subtotal	—	—	—	—

Dinner	Pro	Fat	Carb	Pts or Cal
_____	—	—	—	—
_____	—	—	—	—
_____	—	—	—	—
_____	—	—	—	—
_____	—	—	—	—
Subtotal	—	—	—	—

Snacks	Pro	Fat	Carb	Pts or Cal
_____	—	—	—	—
_____	—	—	—	—
_____	—	—	—	—
Day's Total	—	—	—	—

Date _____   **My Weight** _____   **Weather** _____

Heart rate:
Resting: ____   Max: ____

My goals:
Weight: ____   Heart rate (max) ____

My mood is
❑ Happy   ❑ Ordinary   ❑ Sad

My current state of mind is (check all that apply)
❑ Angry ❑ Frustrated ❑ Determined ❑ Anxious ❑ Not feeling well ❑ Tired
❑ Optimistic ❑ Stressed ❑ Other

I slept
❑ Soundly   ❑ Average   ❑ Below average   ❑ Not at all

Exercise was
❑ Light   ❑ Less than 10 min.
❑ Medium   ❑ 10–30 min.
❑ Intense   ❑ 30–60 min.

I need to pay more attention to _____

_____

_____

_____

_____

My Food Journal

Date _____   My Weight _____   Weather _____

Water ☐☐☐☐   I took my vitamin   ☐
      ☐☐☐☐   Other supplements   ☐

Food Diary

Breakfast	Pro	Fat	Carb	Pts or Cal
_____	—	—	—	—
_____	—	—	—	—
_____	—	—	—	—
_____	—	—	—	—
_____	—	—	—	—
Subtotal	—	—	—	—

Lunch	Pro	Fat	Carb	Pts or Cal
_____	—	—	—	—
_____	—	—	—	—
_____	—	—	—	—
_____	—	—	—	—
_____	—	—	—	—
Subtotal	—	—	—	—

Dinner	Pro	Fat	Carb	Pts or Cal
_____	—	—	—	—
_____	—	—	—	—
_____	—	—	—	—
_____	—	—	—	—
_____	—	—	—	—
Subtotal	—	—	—	—

Snacks	Pro	Fat	Carb	Pts or Cal
_____	—	—	—	—
_____	—	—	—	—
_____	—	—	—	—
Day's Total	—	—	—	—

Date _____   **My Weight** _____   **Weather** _____

Heart rate:
Resting: _____   Max: _____

My goals:
Weight: _____   Heart rate (max) _____

My mood is
❑ Happy   ❑ Ordinary   ❑ Sad

My current state of mind is (check all that apply)
❑ Angry ❑ Frustrated ❑ Determined ❑ Anxious ❑ Not feeling well ❑ Tired
❑ Optimistic ❑ Stressed ❑ Other

I slept
❑ Soundly   ❑ Average   ❑ Below average   ❑ Not at all

Exercise was
❑ Light   ❑ Less than 10 min.
❑ Medium   ❑ 10–30 min.
❑ Intense   ❑ 30–60 min.

I need to pay more attention to _____

_____

_____

_____

_____

My Food Journal

Date _____ **My Weight** _____ **Weather** _____

Water ☐☐☐☐   I took my vitamin   ☐
☐☐☐☐   Other supplements   ☐

Food Diary

Breakfast	Pro	Fat	Carb	Pts or Cal
_____	—	—	—	—
_____	—	—	—	—
_____	—	—	—	—
_____	—	—	—	—
Subtotal	—	—	—	—

Lunch	Pro	Fat	Carb	Pts or Cal
_____	—	—	—	—
_____	—	—	—	—
_____	—	—	—	—
_____	—	—	—	—
Subtotal	—	—	—	—

Dinner	Pro	Fat	Carb	Pts or Cal
_____	—	—	—	—
_____	—	—	—	—
_____	—	—	—	—
Subtotal	—	—	—	—

Snacks	Pro	Fat	Carb	Pts or Cal
_____	—	—	—	—
_____	—	—	—	—
Day's Total	—	—	—	—

Date _____   **My Weight** _____   **Weather** _____

Heart rate:
Resting: _____   Max: _____

My goals:
Weight: _____   Heart rate (max) _____

My mood is
❑ Happy   ❑ Ordinary   ❑ Sad

My current state of mind is (check all that apply)
❑ Angry ❑ Frustrated ❑ Determined ❑ Anxious ❑ Not feeling well ❑ Tired
❑ Optimistic ❑ Stressed ❑ Other

I slept
❑ Soundly   ❑ Average   ❑ Below average   ❑ Not at all

Exercise was
❑ Light   ❑ Less than 10 min.
❑ Medium   ❑ 10–30 min.
❑ Intense   ❑ 30–60 min.

I need to pay more attention to _____

_____

_____

_____

_____

My Food Journal

Date _____   My Weight _____   Weather _____

Water ❏ ❏ ❏ ❏   I took my vitamin   ❏
      ❏ ❏ ❏ ❏   Other supplements   ❏

Food Diary

Breakfast	Pro	Fat	Carb	Pts or Cal
_____	―	―	―	―
_____	―	―	―	―
_____	―	―	―	―
_____	―	―	―	―
_____	―	―	―	―
Subtotal	―	―	―	―

Lunch	Pro	Fat	Carb	Pts or Cal
_____	―	―	―	―
_____	―	―	―	―
_____	―	―	―	―
_____	―	―	―	―
_____	―	―	―	―
Subtotal	―	―	―	―

Dinner	Pro	Fat	Carb	Pts or Cal
_____	―	―	―	―
_____	―	―	―	―
_____	―	―	―	―
_____	―	―	―	―
Subtotal	―	―	―	―

Snacks	Pro	Fat	Carb	Pts or Cal
_____	―	―	―	―
_____	―	―	―	―
_____	―	―	―	―
Day's Total	―	―	―	―

Date _____   **My Weight** _____   **Weather** _____

Heart rate:
Resting: ____   Max: ____

My goals:
Weight: ____   Heart rate (max) ____

My mood is
❏ Happy   ❏ Ordinary   ❏ Sad

My current state of mind is (check all that apply)
❏ Angry ❏ Frustrated ❏ Determined ❏ Anxious ❏ Not feeling well ❏ Tired
❏ Optimistic ❏ Stressed ❏ Other

I slept
❏ Soundly ❏ Average ❏ Below average ❏ Not at all

Exercise was
❏ Light   ❏ Less than 10 min.
❏ Medium   ❏ 10–30 min.
❏ Intense   ❏ 30–60 min.

I need to pay more attention to _____

_____

_____

_____

_____

My Food Journal

Date _____   My Weight _____   Weather _____

Water ☐☐☐☐   I took my vitamin ☐
      ☐☐☐☐   Other supplements ☐

Food Diary

Breakfast	Pro	Fat	Carb	Pts or Cal
_____	—	—	—	—
_____	—	—	—	—
_____	—	—	—	—
_____	—	—	—	—
_____	—	—	—	—
Subtotal	—	—	—	—

Lunch	Pro	Fat	Carb	Pts or Cal
_____	—	—	—	—
_____	—	—	—	—
_____	—	—	—	—
_____	—	—	—	—
_____	—	—	—	—
Subtotal	—	—	—	—

Dinner	Pro	Fat	Carb	Pts or Cal
_____	—	—	—	—
_____	—	—	—	—
_____	—	—	—	—
_____	—	—	—	—
Subtotal	—	—	—	—

Snacks	Pro	Fat	Carb	Pts or Cal
_____	—	—	—	—
_____	—	—	—	—
_____	—	—	—	—
Day's Total	—	—	—	—

Date _____   **My Weight** _____   **Weather** _____

Heart rate:
Resting: _____   Max: _____

My goals:
Weight: _____   Heart rate (max) _____

My mood is
❏ Happy   ❏ Ordinary   ❏ Sad

My current state of mind is (check all that apply)
❏ Angry ❏ Frustrated ❏ Determined ❏ Anxious ❏ Not feeling well ❏ Tired
❏ Optimistic ❏ Stressed ❏ Other

I slept
❏ Soundly ❏ Average ❏ Below average ❏ Not at all

Exercise was
❏ Light   ❏ Less than 10 min.
❏ Medium   ❏ 10–30 min.
❏ Intense   ❏ 30–60 min.

I need to pay more attention to _____

_____

_____

_____

My Food Journal

Date _____   My Weight _____   Weather _____

Water ☐☐☐☐   I took my vitamin   ☐
       ☐☐☐☐   Other supplements   ☐

Food Diary

Breakfast	Pro	Fat	Carb	Pts or Cal
_____	—	—	—	—
_____	—	—	—	—
_____	—	—	—	—
_____	—	—	—	—
_____	—	—	—	—
Subtotal	—	—	—	—

Lunch	Pro	Fat	Carb	Pts or Cal
_____	—	—	—	—
_____	—	—	—	—
_____	—	—	—	—
_____	—	—	—	—
_____	—	—	—	—
Subtotal	—	—	—	—

Dinner	Pro	Fat	Carb	Pts or Cal
_____	—	—	—	—
_____	—	—	—	—
_____	—	—	—	—
_____	—	—	—	—
_____	—	—	—	—
Subtotal	—	—	—	—

Snacks	Pro	Fat	Carb	Pts or Cal
_____	—	—	—	—
_____	—	—	—	—
_____	—	—	—	—
Day's Total	—	—	—	—

Date _____   **My Weight** _____   **Weather** _____

Heart rate:
Resting: _____   Max: _____

My goals:
Weight: _____   Heart rate (max) _____

My mood is
❏ Happy   ❏ Ordinary   ❏ Sad

My current state of mind is (check all that apply)
❏ Angry ❏ Frustrated ❏ Determined ❏ Anxious ❏ Not feeling well ❏ Tired
❏ Optimistic ❏ Stressed ❏ Other

I slept
❏ Soundly ❏ Average ❏ Below average ❏ Not at all

Exercise was
❏ Light   ❏ Less than 10 min.
❏ Medium   ❏ 10–30 min.
❏ Intense   ❏ 30–60 min.

I need to pay more attention to _____

_____

_____

_____

_____

My Food Journal

Date _____   My Weight _____   Weather _____

Water ☐☐☐☐   I took my vitamin   ☐
      ☐☐☐☐   Other supplements   ☐

Food Diary

Breakfast	Pro	Fat	Carb	Pts or Cal
_____	—	—	—	—
_____	—	—	—	—
_____	—	—	—	—
_____	—	—	—	—
_____	—	—	—	—
Subtotal	—	—	—	—

Lunch	Pro	Fat	Carb	Pts or Cal
_____	—	—	—	—
_____	—	—	—	—
_____	—	—	—	—
_____	—	—	—	—
_____	—	—	—	—
Subtotal	—	—	—	—

Dinner	Pro	Fat	Carb	Pts or Cal
_____	—	—	—	—
_____	—	—	—	—
_____	—	—	—	—
_____	—	—	—	—
_____	—	—	—	—
Subtotal	—	—	—	—

Snacks	Pro	Fat	Carb	Pts or Cal
_____	—	—	—	—
_____	—	—	—	—
_____	—	—	—	—
Day's Total	—	—	—	—

Date _____   **My Weight** _____   **Weather** _____

Heart rate:
Resting: ____   Max: ____

My goals:
Weight: ____   Heart rate (max) ____

My mood is
❏ Happy   ❏ Ordinary   ❏ Sad

My current state of mind is (check all that apply)
❏ Angry ❏ Frustrated ❏ Determined ❏ Anxious ❏ Not feeling well ❏ Tired
❏ Optimistic ❏ Stressed ❏ Other

I slept
❏ Soundly   ❏ Average   ❏ Below average   ❏ Not at all

Exercise was
❏ Light   ❏ Less than 10 min.
❏ Medium   ❏ 10–30 min.
❏ Intense   ❏ 30–60 min.

I need to pay more attention to _____

_____

_____

_____

_____

My Food Journal

Date _____   My Weight _____   Weather _____

Water ☐ ☐ ☐ ☐   I took my vitamin   ☐
      ☐ ☐ ☐ ☐   Other supplements   ☐

Food Diary

Breakfast	Pro	Fat	Carb	Pts or Cal
_____	—	—	—	—
_____	—	—	—	—
_____	—	—	—	—
_____	—	—	—	—
_____	—	—	—	—
Subtotal	—	—	—	—

Lunch	Pro	Fat	Carb	Pts or Cal
_____	—	—	—	—
_____	—	—	—	—
_____	—	—	—	—
_____	—	—	—	—
_____	—	—	—	—
Subtotal	—	—	—	—

Dinner	Pro	Fat	Carb	Pts or Cal
_____	—	—	—	—
_____	—	—	—	—
_____	—	—	—	—
_____	—	—	—	—
_____	—	—	—	—
Subtotal	—	—	—	—

Snacks	Pro	Fat	Carb	Pts or Cal
_____	—	—	—	—
_____	—	—	—	—
_____	—	—	—	—
Day's Total	—	—	—	—

Date _____   **My Weight** _____   **Weather** _____

Heart rate:
Resting: ____   Max: ____

My goals:
Weight: ____   Heart rate (max) ____

My mood is
❏ Happy   ❏ Ordinary   ❏ Sad

My current state of mind is (check all that apply)
❏ Angry ❏ Frustrated ❏ Determined ❏ Anxious ❏ Not feeling well ❏ Tired
❏ Optimistic ❏ Stressed ❏ Other

I slept
❏ Soundly   ❏ Average   ❏ Below average   ❏ Not at all

Exercise was
❏ Light   ❏ Less than 10 min.
❏ Medium   ❏ 10–30 min.
❏ Intense   ❏ 30–60 min.

I need to pay more attention to _____

_____

_____

_____

My Food Journal

Date _____   My Weight _____   Weather _____

Water ☐ ☐ ☐ ☐   I took my vitamin   ☐
      ☐ ☐ ☐ ☐   Other supplements   ☐

Food Diary

Breakfast	Pro	Fat	Carb	Pts or Cal
_____	—	—	—	—
_____	—	—	—	—
_____	—	—	—	—
_____	—	—	—	—
_____	—	—	—	—
Subtotal	—	—	—	—

Lunch	Pro	Fat	Carb	Pts or Cal
_____	—	—	—	—
_____	—	—	—	—
_____	—	—	—	—
_____	—	—	—	—
_____	—	—	—	—
Subtotal	—	—	—	—

Dinner	Pro	Fat	Carb	Pts or Cal
_____	—	—	—	—
_____	—	—	—	—
_____	—	—	—	—
_____	—	—	—	—
_____	—	—	—	—
Subtotal	—	—	—	—

Snacks	Pro	Fat	Carb	Pts or Cal
_____	—	—	—	—
_____	—	—	—	—
_____	—	—	—	—
Day's Total	—	—	—	—

Date _____   **My Weight** _____   **Weather** _____

Heart rate:
Resting: ____   Max: ____

My goals:
Weight: ____   Heart rate (max) ____

My mood is
❑ Happy   ❑ Ordinary   ❑ Sad

My current state of mind is (check all that apply)
❑ Angry ❑ Frustrated ❑ Determined ❑ Anxious ❑ Not feeling well ❑ Tired
❑ Optimistic ❑ Stressed ❑ Other

I slept
❑ Soundly   ❑ Average   ❑ Below average   ❑ Not at all

Exercise was
❑ Light   ❑ Less than 10 min.
❑ Medium   ❑ 10–30 min.
❑ Intense   ❑ 30–60 min.

I need to pay more attention to _____

_____

_____

_____

_____

My Food Journal

Date _____   My Weight _____   Weather _____

Water ❑❑❑❑   I took my vitamin   ❑
      ❑❑❑❑   Other supplements   ❑

Food Diary

Breakfast	Pro	Fat	Carb	Pts or Cal
_____	___	___	___	___
_____	___	___	___	___
_____	___	___	___	___
_____	___	___	___	___
	___	___	___	___
Subtotal	___	___	___	___

Lunch	Pro	Fat	Carb	Pts or Cal
_____	___	___	___	___
_____	___	___	___	___
_____	___	___	___	___
_____	___	___	___	___
	___	___	___	___
Subtotal	___	___	___	___

Dinner	Pro	Fat	Carb	Pts or Cal
_____	___	___	___	___
_____	___	___	___	___
_____	___	___	___	___
_____	___	___	___	___
	___	___	___	___
Subtotal	___	___	___	___

Snacks	Pro	Fat	Carb	Pts or Cal
_____	___	___	___	___
_____	___	___	___	___
	___	___	___	___
Day's Total	___	___	___	___

Date _____   **My Weight** _____   **Weather** _____

Heart rate:
Resting: ____   Max: ____

My goals:
Weight: ____   Heart rate (max) ____

My mood is
❏ Happy   ❏ Ordinary   ❏ Sad

My current state of mind is (check all that apply)
❏ Angry ❏ Frustrated ❏ Determined ❏ Anxious ❏ Not feeling well ❏ Tired
❏ Optimistic ❏ Stressed ❏ Other

I slept
❏ Soundly   ❏ Average   ❏ Below average   ❏ Not at all

Exercise was
❏ Light   ❏ Less than 10 min.
❏ Medium   ❏ 10–30 min.
❏ Intense   ❏ 30–60 min.

I need to pay more attention to _____

_____

_____

_____

_____

My Food Journal

Date _____ My Weight _____ Weather _____

Water ☐ ☐ ☐ ☐   I took my vitamin   ☐
☐ ☐ ☐ ☐   Other supplements   ☐

Food Diary

Breakfast	Pro	Fat	Carb	Pts or Cal
_____	—	—	—	—
_____	—	—	—	—
_____	—	—	—	—
_____	—	—	—	—
Subtotal	—	—	—	—

Lunch	Pro	Fat	Carb	Pts or Cal
_____	—	—	—	—
_____	—	—	—	—
_____	—	—	—	—
_____	—	—	—	—
_____	—	—	—	—
Subtotal	—	—	—	—

Dinner	Pro	Fat	Carb	Pts or Cal
_____	—	—	—	—
_____	—	—	—	—
_____	—	—	—	—
_____	—	—	—	—
Subtotal	—	—	—	—

Snacks	Pro	Fat	Carb	Pts or Cal
_____	—	—	—	—
_____	—	—	—	—
Day's Total	—	—	—	—

Date _____   **My Weight** _____   **Weather** _____

Heart rate:
Resting: ____   Max: ____

My goals:
Weight: ____   Heart rate (max) ____

My mood is
❑ Happy ❑ Ordinary ❑ Sad

My current state of mind is (check all that apply)
❑ Angry ❑ Frustrated ❑ Determined ❑ Anxious ❑ Not feeling well ❑ Tired
❑ Optimistic ❑ Stressed ❑ Other

I slept
❑ Soundly ❑ Average ❑ Below average ❑ Not at all

Exercise was
❑ Light   ❑ Less than 10 min.
❑ Medium   ❑ 10–30 min.
❑ Intense   ❑ 30–60 min.

I need to pay more attention to _____

_____

_____

_____

My Food Journal

Date _____   My Weight _____   Weather _____

Water ❑ ❑ ❑ ❑   I took my vitamin   ❑
          ❑ ❑ ❑ ❑   Other supplements   ❑

Food Diary

Breakfast	Pro	Fat	Carb	Pts or Cal
_____	___	___	___	___
_____	___	___	___	___
_____	___	___	___	___
_____	___	___	___	___
_____	___	___	___	___
Subtotal	___	___	___	___

Lunch	Pro	Fat	Carb	Pts or Cal
_____	___	___	___	___
_____	___	___	___	___
_____	___	___	___	___
_____	___	___	___	___
_____	___	___	___	___
Subtotal	___	___	___	___

Dinner	Pro	Fat	Carb	Pts or Cal
_____	___	___	___	___
_____	___	___	___	___
_____	___	___	___	___
_____	___	___	___	___
_____	___	___	___	___
Subtotal	___	___	___	___

Snacks	Pro	Fat	Carb	Pts or Cal
_____	___	___	___	___
_____	___	___	___	___
_____	___	___	___	___
Day's Total	___	___	___	___

Date _____   **My Weight** _____   **Weather** _____

Heart rate:
Resting: ____   Max: ____

My goals:
Weight: ____   Heart rate (max) ____

My mood is
❏ Happy   ❏ Ordinary   ❏ Sad

My current state of mind is (check all that apply)
❏ Angry ❏ Frustrated ❏ Determined ❏ Anxious ❏ Not feeling well ❏ Tired
❏ Optimistic ❏ Stressed ❏ Other

I slept
❏ Soundly   ❏ Average   ❏ Below average   ❏ Not at all

Exercise was
❏ Light   ❏ Less than 10 min.
❏ Medium   ❏ 10–30 min.
❏ Intense   ❏ 30–60 min.

I need to pay more attention to _____

_____

_____

_____

_____

My Food Journal

Date _____   **My Weight** _____   **Weather** _____

Water ☐ ☐ ☐ ☐   I took my vitamin   ☐
      ☐ ☐ ☐ ☐   Other supplements   ☐

Food Diary

Breakfast	Pro	Fat	Carb	Pts or Cal
_____	—	—	—	—
_____	—	—	—	—
_____	—	—	—	—
_____	—	—	—	—
Subtotal	—	—	—	—

Lunch	Pro	Fat	Carb	Pts or Cal
_____	—	—	—	—
_____	—	—	—	—
_____	—	—	—	—
_____	—	—	—	—
Subtotal	—	—	—	—

Dinner	Pro	Fat	Carb	Pts or Cal
_____	—	—	—	—
_____	—	—	—	—
_____	—	—	—	—
_____	—	—	—	—
Subtotal	—	—	—	—

Snacks	Pro	Fat	Carb	Pts or Cal
_____	—	—	—	—
_____	—	—	—	—
_____	—	—	—	—
Day's Total	—	—	—	—

Date _____   **My Weight** _____   **Weather** _____

Heart rate:
Resting: ____   Max: ____

My goals:
Weight: ____   Heart rate (max) ____

My mood is
❑ Happy   ❑ Ordinary   ❑ Sad

My current state of mind is (check all that apply)
❑ Angry ❑ Frustrated ❑ Determined ❑ Anxious ❑ Not feeling well ❑ Tired
❑ Optimistic ❑ Stressed ❑ Other

I slept
❑ Soundly   ❑ Average   ❑ Below average   ❑ Not at all

Exercise was
❑ Light   ❑ Less than 10 min.
❑ Medium   ❑ 10–30 min.
❑ Intense   ❑ 30–60 min.

I need to pay more attention to _____

_____

_____

_____

_____

Graphing My Weight Loss

Fill in the date you weigh yourself at the bottom of the graph and put a dot on the grid opposite the number nearest your actual weight to mark your daily, weekly, or periodic weigh-ins. As you weigh yourself, join the dots; this visual aid makes it easy to pinpoint stalls and other problems. You might want to photocopy this page before you start using it; you might find as you go along that you may need more space.

Graphing My Weight Loss

Weight (in Pounds)															
250															
245															
240															
235															
230															
225															
220															
215															
210															
205															
200															
195															
190															
185															
180															
175															
170															
165															
160															
155															
150															
Date															

Appendix C

Nutritive Table of Foods

	Portion	Calories (kcal)	Protein (g)	Total Fat (g)	Carbo-hydrate (g)	Total Dietary Fiber (g)
Beverages						
Alcoholic						
Beer						
Regular	12 fl. oz.	146	1	0	13	0.7
Light	12 fl. oz.	99	1	0	5	0.0
Gin, rum, vodka, whiskey						
80 proof	1.5 fl. oz.	97	0	0	0	0.0
86 proof	1.5 fl. oz.	105	0	0	Tr	0.0
90 proof	1.5 fl. oz.	110	0	0	0	0.0
Liqueur, coffee, 53 proof	1.5 fl. oz.	175	Tr	Tr	24	0.0
Mixed drinks, prepared from recipe						
Daiquiri	2 fl. oz.	112	Tr	Tr	4	0.0
Piña colada	4.5 fl. oz.	262	1	3	40	0.8
Wine						
Dessert						
Dry	3.5 fl. oz.	130	Tr	0	4	0.0
Sweet	3.5 fl. oz.	158	Tr	0	12	0.0
Table						
Red	3.5 fl. oz.	74	Tr	0	2	0.0
White	3.5 fl. oz.	70	Tr	0	1	0.0

	Portion	Calories (kcal)	Protein (g)	Total Fat (g)	Carbo-hydrate (g)	Total Dietary Fiber (g)
Carbonated*						
Club soda	12 fl. oz.	0	0	0	0	0.0
Cola type	12 fl. oz.	152	0	0	38	0.0
Diet, sweetened with aspartame						
Cola	12 fl. oz.	4	Tr	0	Tr	0.0
Other than cola or pepper type	12 fl. oz.	0	Tr	0	0	0.0
Ginger ale	12 fl. oz.	124	0	0	32	0.0
Grape	12 fl. oz.	160	0	0	42	0.0
Lemon lime	12 fl. oz.	147	0	0	38	0.0
Orange	12 fl. oz.	179	0	0	46	0.0
Pepper type	12 fl. oz.	151	0	Tr	38	0.0
Root beer	12 fl. oz.	152	0	0	39	0.0
Chocolate flavored beverage mix						
Powder	2-3 heaping tsp.	75	1	1	20	1.3
Prepared with milk	1 cup	226	9	9	31	1.3
Cocoa powder containing nonfat dry milk						
Powder	3 heaping tsp.	102	3	1	22	0.3
Prepared (6 oz. water plus 1 oz. powder)	1 serving	103	3	1	22	2.5
Powder containing nonfat dry milk and aspartame						
Powder	½-oz. envelope	48	4	Tr	9	0.4
Prepared (6 oz. water plus 1 envelope mix)	1 serving	48	4	Tr	8	0.4
Coffee						
Brewed	6 fl. oz.	4	Tr	0	1	0.0
Espresso	2 fl. oz.	5	Tr	Tr	1	0.0
Instant, prepared (1 rounded tsp. powder plus 6 fl. oz. water)	6 fl. oz.	4	Tr	0	1	0.0

Mineral content varies depending on water source.

	Portion	Calories (kcal)	Protein (g)	Total Fat (g)	Carbo-hydrate (g)	Total Dietary Fiber (g)
Fruit drinks, non-carbonated, canned or bottled, with added ascorbic acid						
Cranberry juice cocktail	8 fl. oz.	144	0	Tr	36	0.3
Fruit punch drink	8 fl. oz.	117	0	0	30	0.2
Grape drink	8 fl. oz.	113	0	0	29	0.0
Pineapple grapefruit juice drink	8 fl. oz.	118	1	Tr	29	0.3
Pineapple orange juice drink	8 fl. oz.	125	3	0	30	0.3
Lemonade						
Frozen concentrate, prepared	8 fl. oz.	99	Tr	0	26	0.2
Powder, prepared with water						
Regular	8 fl. oz.	112	0	0	29	0.0
Low calorie, sweetened with aspartame	8 fl. oz.	5	0	0	1	0.0
Malted milk, with added nutrients						
Chocolate						
Powder	3 heaping tsp.	75	1	1	18	0.2
Prepared	1 cup	225	9	9	29	0.3
Natural						
Powder	4-5 heaping tsp.	80	2	1	17	0.1
Prepared	1 cup	231	10	9	28	0.0
Milk and milk beverages (see Dairy products)						
Rice beverage, canned (RICE DREAM)	1 cup	120	Tr	2	25	0.0
Soy milk (see Legumes, nuts, and seeds)						

	Portion	Calories (kcal)	Protein (g)	Total Fat (g)	Carbo-hydrate (g)	Total Dietary Fiber (g)
Tea						
Brewed						
Black	6 fl. oz.	2	0	0	1	0.0
Chamomile	6 fl. oz.	2	0	0	Tr	0.0
Other than chamomile	6 fl. oz.	2	0	0	Tr	0.0
Instant, powder, prepared						
Unsweetened	8 fl. oz.	2	0	0	Tr	0.0
Sweetened, lemon flavor	8 fl. oz.	88	Tr	0	22	0.0
Sweetened with saccharin, lemon flavor	8 fl. oz.	5	0	0	1	0.0
Water, tap	8 fl. oz.	0	0	0	0	0.0

Dairy products

	Portion	Calories (kcal)	Protein (g)	Total Fat (g)	Carbo-hydrate (g)	Total Dietary Fiber (g)
Butter (see Fats and oils)						
Cheese						
Natural						
Blue	1 oz.	100	6	8	1	0.0
Camembert (3 wedges per 4-oz. container)	1 wedge	114	8	9	Tr	0.0
Cheddar						
Cut pieces	1 oz.	114	7	9	Tr	0.0
	1 cubic inch	68	4	6	Tr	0.0
Shredded	1 cup	455	28	37	1	0.0
Cottage						
Creamed (4% fat)						
Large curd	1 cup	233	28	10	6	0.0
Small curd	1 cup	217	26	9	6	0.0
With fruit	1 cup	279	22	8	30	0.0
Low fat (2%)	1 cup	203	31	4	8	0.0
Low fat (1%)	1 cup	164	28	2	6	0.0
Uncreamed (dry curd, less than ½ % fat)	1 cup	123	25	1	3	0.0

	Portion	Calories (kcal)	Protein (g)	Total Fat (g)	Carbo-hydrate (g)	Total Dietary Fiber (g)
Cream						
Regular	1 oz.	99	2	10	1	0.0
	1 TB.	51	1	5	Tr	0.0
Low fat	1 TB.	35	2	3	1	0.0
Fat free	1 TB.	15	2	Tr	1	0.0
Feta	1 oz.	75	4	6	1	0.0
Low fat, cheddar or colby	1 oz.	49	7	2	1	0.0
Mozzarella, made with						
Whole milk	1 oz.	80	6	6	1	0.0
Part skim milk (low moisture)	1 oz.	79	8	5	1	0.0
Muenster	1 oz.	104	7	9	Tr	0.0
Neufchatel	1 oz.	74	3	7	1	0.0
Parmesan, grated	1 cup	456	42	30	4	0.0
	1 TB.	23	2	2	Tr	0.0
	1 oz.	129	12	9	1	0.0
Provolone	1 oz.	100	7	8	1	0.0
Ricotta, made with						
Whole milk	1 cup	428	28	32	7	0.0
Part skim milk	1 cup	340	28	19	13	0.0
Swiss	1 oz.	107	8	8	1	0.0
Pasteurized process cheese						
American						
Regular	1 oz.	106	6	9	Tr	0.0
Fat free	1 slice	31	5	Tr	3	0.0
Swiss	1 oz.	95	7	7	1	0.0
Pasteurized process cheese food, American	1 oz.	93	6	7	2	0.0
Pasteurized process cheese spread, American	1 oz.	82	5	6	2	0.0
Cream, sweet						
Half and half (cream and milk)	1 cup	315	7	28	10	0.0
	1 TB.	20	Tr	2	1	0.0
Light, coffee, or table	1 cup	469	6	46	9	0.0
	1 TB.	29	Tr	3	1	0.0

	Portion	Calories (kcal)	Protein (g)	Total Fat (g)	Carbo-hydrate (g)	Total Dietary Fiber (g)
Whipping, unwhipped (volume about double when whipped)						
Light	1 cup	699	5	74	7	0.0
	1 TB.	44	Tr	5	Tr	0.0
Heavy	1 cup	821	5	88	7	0.0
	1 TB.	52	Tr	6	Tr	0.0
Whipped topping (pressurized)	1 cup	154	2	13	7	0.0
	1 TB.	8	Tr	1	Tr	0.0
Cream, sour						
Regular	1 cup	493	7	48	10	0.0
	1 TB.	26	Tr	3	1	0.0
Reduced fat	1 TB.	20	Tr	2	1	0.0
Fat free	1 TB.	12	Tr	0	2	0.0
Cream product, imitation (made with vegetable fat)						
Sweet creamer						
Liquid (frozen)	1 TB.	20	Tr	1	2	0.0
Powdered	1 tsp	11	Tr	1	1	0.0
Whipped topping						
Frozen	1 cup	239	1	19	17	0.0
	1 TB.	13	Tr	1	1	0.0
Powdered, prepared with whole milk	1 cup	151	3	10	13	0.0
	1 TB.	8	Tr	Tr	1	0.0
Pressurized	1 cup	184	1	16	11	0.0
	1 TB.	11	Tr	1	1	0.0
Sour dressing (filled cream type, nonbutterfat)	1 cup	417	8	39	11	0.0
	1 TB.	21	Tr	2	1	0.0
Frozen dessert						
Frozen yogurt, soft serve						
Chocolate	½ cup	115	3	4	18	1.6
Vanilla	½ cup	114	3	4	17	0.0
Ice cream						
Regular						
Chocolate	½ cup	143	3	7	19	0.8
Vanilla	½ cup	133	2	7	16	0.0

	Portion	Calories (kcal)	Protein (g)	Total Fat (g)	Carbo-hydrate (g)	Total Dietary Fiber (g)
Light (50% reduced fat), vanilla	½ cup	92	3	3	15	0.0
Premium low fat, chocolate	½ cup	113	3	2	22	0.7
Rich, vanilla	½ cup	178	3	12	17	0.0
Soft serve, french vanilla	½ cup	185	4	11	19	0.0
Sherbet, orange	½ cup	102	1	1	22	0.0
Milk						
Fluid, no milk solids added						
Whole (3.3% fat)	1 cup	150	8	8	11	0.0
Reduced fat (2%)	1 cup	121	8	5	12	0.0
Lowfat (1%)	1 cup	102	8	3	12	0.0
Nonfat (skim)	1 cup	86	8	Tr	12	0.0
Buttermilk	1 cup	99	8	2	12	0.0
Canned						
Condensed, sweetened	1 cup	982	24	27	166	0.0
Evaporated						
Whole milk	1 cup	339	17	19	25	0.0
Skim milk	1 cup	199	19	1	29	0.0
Dried						
Buttermilk	1 cup	464	41	7	59	0.0
Nonfat, instant, with added vitamin A	1 cup	244	24	Tr	35	0.0
Milk beverage						
Chocolate milk (commercial)						
Whole	1 cup	208	8	8	26	2.0
Reduced fat (2%)	1 cup	179	8	5	26	1.3
Lowfat (1%)	1 cup	158	8	3	26	1.3
Eggnog (commercial)	1 cup	342	10	19	34	0.0
Milk shake, thick						
Chocolate	10.6 fl. oz.	356	9	8	63	0.9
Vanilla	11 fl. oz.	350	12	9	56	0.0
Sherbet (see Dairy products, Frozen dessert)						

	Portion	Calories (kcal)	Protein (g)	Total Fat (g)	Carbo-hydrate (g)	Total Dietary Fiber (g)
Yogurt						
With added milk solids						
Made with lowfat milk						
Fruit flavored	8-oz. container	231	10	2	43	0.0
Plain	8-oz. container	144	12	4	16	0.0
Made with nonfat milk						
Fruit flavored	8-oz. container	213	10	Tr	43	0.0
Plain	8-oz. container	127	13	Tr	17	0.0
Without added milk solids						
Made with whole milk, plain	8-oz. container	139	8	7	11	0.0
Made with nonfat milk, low calorie sweetener, vanilla or lemon flavor	8-oz. container	98	9	Tr	17	0.0
Eggs						
Raw						
Whole	1 medium	66	5	4	1	0.0
	1 large	75	6	5	1	0.0
	1 extra large	86	7	6	1	0.0
White	1 large	17	4	0	Tr	0.0
Yolk	1 large	59	3	5	Tr	0.0
Cooked, whole fried, in margarine, with salt	1 large	92	6	7	1	0.0
Hard cooked, shell removed	1 large	78	6	5	1	0.0
	1 cup chopped	211	17	14	2	0.0
Poached, with salt	1 large	75	6	5	1	0.0
Scrambled, in margarine, with whole milk, salt	1 large	101	7	7	1	0.0
Egg substitute, liquid	¼ cup	53	8	2	Tr	0.0
Fats and oils						
Butter (4 sticks per lb.)						
Salted	1 stick	813	1	92	Tr	0.0
	1 TB.	102	Tr	12	Tr	0.0
	1 tsp.	36	Tr	4	Tr	0.0

	Portion	Calories (kcal)	Protein (g)	Total Fat (g)	Carbo-hydrate (g)	Total Dietary Fiber (g)
Unsalted	1 stick	813	1	92	Tr	0.0
Lard	1 cup	1,849	0	205	0	0.0
	1 TB.	115	0	13	0	0.0
Margarine, vitamin A-fortified, salt added						
Regular (about 80% fat)						
Hard (4 sticks per lb.)	1 stick	815	1	91	1	0.0
	1 TB.	101	Tr	11	Tr	0.0
	1 tsp.	34	Tr	4	Tr	0.0
Soft	1 cup	1,626	2	183	1	0.0
	1 tsp.	34	Tr	4	Tr	0.0
Spread (about 60% fat)						
Hard (4 sticks per lb.)	1 stick	621	1	70	0	0.0
	1 TB.	76	Tr	9	0	0.0
	1 tsp.	26	Tr	3	0	0.0
Soft	1 cup	1,236	1	139	0	0.0
	1 tsp.	26	Tr	3	0	0.0
Spread (about 40% fat)	1 cup	801	1	90	1	0.0
	1 tsp.	17	Tr	2	Tr	0.0
Margarine butter blend	1 stick	811	1	91	1	0.0
	1 TB.	102	Tr	11	Tr	0.0
Oils, salad or cooking						
Canola	1 cup	1,927	0	218	0	0.0
	1 TB.	124	0	14	0	0.0
Corn	1 cup	1,927	0	218	0	0.0
	1 TB.	120	0	14	0	0.0
Olive	1 cup	1,909	0	216	0	0.0
	1 TB.	119	0	14	0	0.0
Peanut	1 cup	1,909	0	216	0	0.0
	1 TB.	119	0	14	0	0.0
Safflower, high oleic	1 cup	1,927	0	218	0	0.0
	1 TB.	120	0	14	0	0.0
Sesame	1 cup	1,927	0	218	0	0.0
	1 TB.	120	0	14	0	0.0
Soybean, hydrogenated	1 cup	1,927	0	218	0	0.0
	1 TB.	120	0	14	0	0.0

	Portion	Calories (kcal)	Protein (g)	Total Fat (g)	Carbo- hydrate (g)	Total Dietary Fiber (g)
Soybean, hydrogenated and cottonseed oil blend	1 cup	1,927	0	218	0	0.0
	1 TB.	120	0	14	0	0.0
Sunflower	1 cup	1,927	0	218	0	0.0
	1 TB.	120	0	14	0	0.0
Salad dressings						
Commercial						
Blue cheese						
Regular	1 TB.	77	1	8	1	0.0
Low calorie	1 TB.	15	1	1	Tr	0.0
Caesar						
Regular	1 TB.	78	Tr	8	Tr	Tr
Low calorie	1 TB.	17	Tr	1	3	Tr
French						
Regular	1 TB.	67	Tr	6	3	0.0
Low calorie	1 TB.	22	Tr	1	4	0.0
Italian						
Regular	1 TB.	69	Tr	7	1	0.0
Low calorie	1 TB.	16	Tr	1	1	Tr
Mayonnaise						
Regular	1 TB.	99	Tr	11	Tr	0.0
Light, cholesterol free	1 TB.	49	Tr	5	1	0.0
Fat free	1 TB.	12	0	Tr	2	0.6
Russian						
Regular	1 TB.	76	Tr	8	2	0.0
Low calorie	1 TB.	23	Tr	1	4	Tr
Thousand Island						
Regular	1 TB.	59	Tr	6	2	0.0
Low calorie	1 TB.	24	Tr	2	2	0.2
Prepared from home recipe						
Cooked, made with margarine	1 TB.	25	1	2	2	0.0
French	1 TB.	88	Tr	10	Tr	0.0
Vinegar and oil	1 TB.	70	0	8	Tr	0.0
Shortening	1 cup	1,812	0	205	0	0.0
(hydrogenated soybean and cottonseed oils)	1 TB.	113	0	13	0	0.0

	Portion	Calories (kcal)	Protein (g)	Total Fat (g)	Carbo-hydrate (g)	Total Dietary Fiber (g)
			Fish and Shellfish			
Catfish, breaded, fried	3 oz.	195	15	11	7	0.6
Clam						
Raw, meat only	3 oz.	63	11	1	2	0.0
	1 medium	11	2	Tr	Tr	0.0
Breaded, fried	¾ cup	451	13	26	39	0.3
Canned, drained solids	3 oz.	126	22	2	4	0.0
	1 cup	237	41	3	8	0.0
Cod						
Baked or broiled	3 oz.	89	20	1	0	0.0
	1 fillet	95	21	1	0	0.0
Canned, solids and liquid	3 oz.	89	19	1	0	0.0
Crab						
Alaska king						
Steamed	1 leg	130	26	2	0	0.0
	3 oz.	82	16	1	0	0.0
Imitation, from surimi	3 oz.	87	10	1	9	0.0
Blue						
Steamed	3 oz.	87	17	2	0	0.0
Canned crabmeat	1 cup	134	28	2	0	0.0
Crab cake, with egg, onion, fried in margarine	1 cake	93	12	5	Tr	0.0
Fish fillet, battered or breaded, fried	1 fillet	211	13	11	15	0.5
Fish stick, breaded,	1 stick (4" × 1" × ½")	76	4	3	7	0.0
frozen, reheated	1 portion (4" × 2" × ½")	155	9	7	14	0.0
Flounder or sole, baked or broiled	3 oz.	99	21	1	0	0.0
	1 fillet	149	31	2	0	0.0
Haddock, baked or broiled	3 oz.	95	21	1	0	0.0
	1 fillet	168	36	1	0	0.0
Halibut, baked or broiled	3 oz.	119	23	2	0	0.0
	½ fillet	223	42	5	0	0.0
Herring, pickled	3 oz.	223	12	15	8	0.0

	Portion	Calories (kcal)	Protein (g)	Total Fat (g)	Carbo-hydrate (g)	Total Dietary Fiber (g)
Lobster, steamed	3 oz.	83	17	1	1	0.0
Ocean perch, baked or broiled	3 oz.	103	20	2	0	0.0
	1 fillet	61	12	1	0	0.0
Oyster						
Raw, meat only	1 cup	169	17	6	10	0.0
	6 medium	57	6	2	3	0.0
Breaded, fried	3 oz.	167	7	11	10	0.2
Pollock, baked or broiled	3 oz.	96	20	1	0	0.0
	1 fillet	68	14	1	0	0.0
Rockfish, baked or broiled	3 oz.	103	20	2	0	0.0
	1 fillet	180	36	3	0	0.0
Roughy, orange, baked or broiled	3 oz.	76	16	1	0	0.0
Salmon						
Baked or broiled (red)	3 oz.	184	23	9	0	0.0
	½ fillet	335	42	17	0	0.0
Canned (pink), solids and liquid (includes bones)	3 oz.	118	17	5	0	0.0
Smoked (chinook)	3 oz.	99	16	4	0	0.0
Sardine, Atlantic, canned in oil, drained solids (includes bones)	3 oz.	177	21	10	0	0.0
Scallop, cooked						
Breaded, fried	6 large	200	17	10	9	0.2
Steamed	3 oz.	95	20	1	3	0.0
Shrimp						
Breaded, fried	3 oz.	206	18	10	10	0.3
	6 large	109	10	6	5	0.2
Canned, drained solids	3 oz.	102	20	2	1	0.0
Swordfish, baked or broiled	3 oz.	132	22	4	0	0.0
	1 piece	164	27	5	0	0.0
Trout, baked or broiled	3 oz.	144	21	6	0	0.0
	1 fillet	120	17	5	0	0.0
Tuna						
Baked or broiled	3 oz.	118	25	1	0	0.0
Canned, drained solids						
Oil pack, chunk light	3 oz.	168	25	7	0	0.0

	Portion	Calories (kcal)	Protein (g)	Total Fat (g)	Carbo-hydrate (g)	Total Dietary Fiber (g)
Water pack, chunk light	3 oz.	99	22	1	0	0.0
Water pack, solid white	3 oz.	109	20	3	0	0.0
Tuna salad: light tuna in oil, pickle relish, mayo-type salad dressing	1 cup	383	33	19	19	0.0

Fruits and fruit juices

Apples						
Raw						
Unpeeled, 2¾" dia (about 3 per lb.)	1 apple	81	Tr	Tr	21	3.7
Peeled, sliced	1 cup	63	Tr	Tr	16	2.1
Dried (sodium bisulfite used to preserve color)	5 rings	78	Tr	Tr	21	2.8
Apple juice, bottled or canned	1 cup	117	Tr	Tr	29	0.2
Apple pie filling, canned	⅛ of 21-oz. can	75	Tr	Tr	19	0.7
Applesauce, canned						
Sweetened	1 cup	194	Tr	Tr	51	3.1
Unsweetened	1 cup	105	Tr	Tr	28	2.9
Apricots						
Raw, without pits (about 12 per lb. with pits)	1 apricot	17	Tr	Tr	4	0.8
Canned, halves, fruit and liquid						
Heavy syrup pack	1 cup	214	1	Tr	55	4.1
Juice pack	1 cup	117	2	Tr	30	3.9
Dried, sulfured	10 halves	83	1	Tr	22	3.2
Apricot nectar, canned, with added ascorbic acid	1 cup	141	1	Tr	36	1.5
Asian pear, raw						
2¼" high × 2½" dia	1 pear	51	1	Tr	13	4.4
3⅜" high × 3" dia	1 pear	116	1	1	29	9.9
Avocados, raw, without skin and seed						
California (about ⅕ whole)	1 oz.	50	1	5	2	1.4
Florida (about ⅒ whole)	1 oz.	32	Tr	3	3	1.5

	Portion	Calories (kcal)	Protein (g)	Total Fat (g)	Carbo-hydrate (g)	Total Dietary Fiber (g)
Bananas, raw						
Whole, medium (7"–7⅞" long)	1 banana	109	1	1	28	2.8
Sliced	1 cup	138	2	1	35	3.6
Blackberries, raw	1 cup	75	1	1	18	7.6
Blueberries						
Raw	1 cup	81	1	1	20	3.9
Frozen, sweetened, thawed	1 cup	186	1	Tr	50	4.8
Cantaloupe (ee Melons)						
Carambola (starfruit), raw						
Whole (3⅝" long)	1 fruit	30	Tr	Tr	7	2.5
Sliced	1 cup	36	1	Tr	8	2.9
Cherries						
Sour, red, pitted, canned, water pack	1 cup	88	2	Tr	22	2.7
Sweet, raw, without pits and stems	10 cherries	49	1	1	11	1.6
Cherry pie filling, canned	⅓ of 21-oz. can	85	Tr	Tr	21	0.4
Cranberries, dried, sweetened	¼ cup	92	Tr	Tr	24	2.5
Cranberry sauce, sweetened, canned (about 8 slices per can)	1 slice	86	Tr	Tr	22	0.6
Dates, without pits						
Whole	5 dates	116	1	Tr	31	3.2
Chopped	1 cup	490	4	1	131	13.4
Figs, dried	2 figs	97	1	Tr	25	4.6
Fruit cocktail, canned, fruit and liquid						
Heavy syrup pack	1 cup	181	1	Tr	47	2.5
Juice pack	1 cup	109	1	Tr	28	2.4
Grapefruit						
Raw, without peel, membrane and seeds (3¼" dia.)						
Pink or red	½ grapefruit	37	1	Tr	9	1.4
White	½ grapefruit	39	1	Tr	10	1.3
Canned, sections with light syrup	1 cup	152	1	Tr	39	1.0

	Portion	Calories (kcal)	Protein (g)	Total Fat (g)	Carbo-hydrate (g)	Total Dietary Fiber (g)
Grapefruit juice						
Raw						
Pink	1 cup	96	1	Tr	23	0.2
White	1 cup	96	1	Tr	23	0.2
Canned						
Unsweetened	1 cup	94	1	Tr	22	0.2
Sweetened	1 cup	115	1	Tr	28	0.3
Frozen concentrate, unsweetened						
Undiluted	6 fl. oz. can	302	4	1	72	0.8
Diluted with 3 parts water by volume	1 cup	101	1	Tr	24	0.2
Grapes, seedless, raw	10 grapes	36	Tr	Tr	9	0.5
	1 cup	114	1	1	28	1.6
Grape juice						
Canned or bottled	1 cup	154	1	Tr	38	0.3
Frozen concentrate, sweetened, with added vitamin C						
Undiluted	6 fl. oz. can	387	1	1	96	0.6
Diluted with 3 parts water by volume	1 cup	128	Tr	Tr	32	0.3
Kiwi fruit, raw, without skin (about 5 per lb. with skin)	1 medium	46	1	Tr	11	2.6
Lemons, raw, without peel (2⅛" dia. with peel)	1 lemon	17	1	Tr	5	1.6
Lemon juice						
Raw (from 2⅛" dia. lemon)	Juice of 1 lemon	12	Tr	0	4	0.2
Canned or bottled, unsweetened	1 cup	51	1	1	16	1.0
	1 TB.	3	Tr	Tr	1	0.1
Lime juice						
Raw (from 2" dia. lime)	juice of 1 lime	10	Tr	Tr	3	0.2
Canned, unsweetened	1 cup	52	1	1	16	1.0
	1 TB.	3	Tr	Tr	1	0.1

	Portion	Calories (kcal)	Protein (g)	Total Fat (g)	Carbo-hydrate (g)	Total Dietary Fiber (g)
Mangos, raw, without skin and seed (about 1 ½ per lb. with skin and seed)						
Whole	1 mango	135	1	1	35	3.7
Sliced	1 cup	107	1	Tr	28	3.0
Melons, raw, without rind and cavity contents						
Cantaloupe (5" dia.)						
Wedge	⅛ melon	24	1	Tr	6	0.6
Cubes	1 cup	56	1	Tr	13	1.3
Honeydew (6"–7" dia.)						
Wedge	⅛ melon	56	1	Tr	15	1.0
Diced (about 20 pieces per cup)	1 cup	60	1	Tr	16	1.0
Mixed fruit, frozen, sweetened, thawed (peach, cherry, raspberry, grape, and boysenberry)	1 cup	245	4	Tr	61	4.8
Nectarines, raw (2½" dia.)	1 nectarine	67	1	1	16	2.2
Oranges, raw						
Whole, without peel and seeds (2⅝" dia.)	1 orange	62	1	Tr	15	3.1
Sections without membranes	1 cup	85	2	Tr	21	4.3
Orange juice						
Raw, all varieties	1 cup	112	2	Tr	26	0.5
	juice from 1 orange	39	1	Tr	9	0.2
Canned, unsweetened	1 cup	105	1	Tr	25	0.5
Chilled (refrigerator case)	1 cup	110	2	1	25	0.5
Frozen concentrate						
Undiluted	6 fl. oz. can	339	5	Tr	81	1.7
Diluted with 3 parts water by volume	1 cup	112	2	Tr	27	0.5
Papayas, raw						
½" cubes	1 cup	55	1	Tr	14	2.5
Whole (5⅛" long × 3" dia.)	1 papaya	119	2	Tr	30	5.5

	Portion	Calories (kcal)	Protein (g)	Total Fat (g)	Carbo-hydrate (g)	Total Dietary Fiber (g)
Peaches						
Raw						
Whole, 2½" dia., pitted (about 4 per lb.)	1 peach	42	1	Tr	11	2.0
Sliced	1 cup	73	1	Tr	19	3.4
Canned, fruit and liquid						
Heavy syrup pack	1 cup	194	1	Tr	52	3.4
	1 half	73	Tr	Tr	20	1.3
Juice pack	1 cup	109	2	Tr	29	3.2
	1 half	43	1	Tr	11	1.3
Dried, sulfured	3 halves	93	1	Tr	24	3.2
Frozen, sliced, sweetened, with added ascorbic acid, thawed	1 cup	235	2	Tr	60	4.5
Pears						
Raw, with skin, cored, 2½" dia.	1 pear	98	1	1	25	4.0
Canned, fruit and liquid						
Heavy syrup pack	1 cup	197	1	Tr	51	4.3
	1 half	56	Tr	Tr	15	1.2
Juice pack	1 cup	124	1	Tr	32	4.0
	1 half	38	Tr	Tr	10	1.2
Pineapple						
Raw, diced	1 cup	76	1	1	19	1.9
Canned, fruit and liquid						
Heavy syrup pack						
Crushed, sliced, or chunks	1 cup	198	1	Tr	51	2.0
Slices (3" dia.)	1 slice	38	Tr	Tr	10	0.4
Juice pack						
Crushed, sliced, or chunks	1 cup	149	1	Tr	39	2.0
Slice (3" dia.)	1 slice	28	Tr	Tr	7	0.4
Pineapple juice, unsweetened, canned	1 cup	140	1	Tr	34	0.5

	Portion	Calories (kcal)	Protein (g)	Total Fat (g)	Carbo-hydrate (g)	Total Dietary Fiber (g)
Plantain, without peel						
Raw	1 medium	218	2	1	57	4.1
Cooked, slices	1 cup	179	1	Tr	48	3.5
Plums						
Raw (2⅛" dia.)	1 plum	36	1	Tr	9	1.0
Canned, purple, fruit and liquid						
Heavy syrup pack	1 cup	230	1	Tr	60	2.6
	1 plum	41	Tr	Tr	11	0.5
Juice pack	1 cup	146	1	Tr	38	2.5
	1 plum	27	Tr	Tr	7	0.5
Prunes, dried, pitted						
Uncooked	5 prunes	100	1	Tr	26	3.0
Stewed, unsweetened, fruit and liquid	1 cup	265	3	1	70	16.4
Prune juice, canned or bottled	1 cup	182	2	Tr	45	2.6
Raisins, seedless						
Cup, not packed	1 cup	435	5	1	115	5.8
Packet, ½ oz. (1½ TB.)	1 packet	42	Tr	Tr	11	0.6
Raspberries						
Raw	1 cup	60	1	1	14	8.4
Frozen, sweetened, thawed	1 cup	258	2	Tr	65	11.0
Rhubarb, frozen, cooked, with sugar	1 cup	278	1	Tr	75	4.8
Strawberries						
Raw, capped						
Large (1⅛" dia.)	1 strawberry	5	Tr	Tr	1	0.4
Medium (1¼" dia.)	1 strawberry	4	Tr	Tr	1	0.3
Sliced	1 cup	50	1	1	12	3.8
Frozen, sweetened, sliced, thawed	1 cup	245	1	Tr	66	4.8
Tangerines						
Raw, without peel and seeds (2⅜" dia.)	1 tangerine	37	1	Tr	9	1.9
Canned (mandarin oranges), light syrup, fruit and liquid	1 cup	154	1	Tr	41	1.8

	Portion	Calories (kcal)	Protein (g)	Total Fat (g)	Carbo-hydrate (g)	Total Dietary Fiber (g)
Tangerine juice, canned, sweetened	1 cup	125	1	Tr	30	0.5
Watermelon, raw (15" long × 7½" dia.)						
Wedge (about 1⁄16 of melon)	1 wedge	92	2	1	21	1.4
Diced	1 cup	49	1	1	11	0.8

Grain products

	Portion	Calories (kcal)	Protein (g)	Total Fat (g)	Carbo-hydrate (g)	Total Dietary Fiber (g)
Bagels, enriched						
Plain	3½" bagel	195	7	1	38	1.6
	4" bagel	245	9	1	48	2.0
Cinnamon raisin	3½" bagel	195	7	1	39	1.6
	4" bagel	244	9	2	49	2.0
Egg	3½" bagel	197	8	1	38	1.6
	4" bagel	247	9	2	47	2.0
Banana bread, prepared from recipe, with margarine	1 slice	196	3	6	33	0.7
Barley, pearled						
Uncooked	1 cup	704	20	2	155	31.2
Cooked	1 cup	193	4	1	44	6.0
Biscuits, plain or buttermilk, enriched						
Prepared from recipe, with 2% milk	2½" biscuit	212	4	10	27	0.9
	4" biscuit	358	7	16	45	1.5
Refrigerated dough, baked						
Regular	2½" biscuit	93	2	4	13	0.4
Lower fat	2¼" biscuit	63	2	1	12	0.4
Breads, enriched						
Cracked wheat	1 slice	65	2	1	12	1.4
Egg bread (challah)	½" slice	115	4	2	19	0.9
French or Vienna (includes sourdough)	½" slice	69	2	1	13	0.8
Indian fry (Navajo) bread	5" bread	296	6	9	48	1.6
	10½" bread	526	11	15	85	2.9
Italian	1 slice	54	2	1	10	0.5

	Portion	Calories (kcal)	Protein (g)	Total Fat (g)	Carbo-hydrate (g)	Total Dietary Fiber (g)
Mixed grain						
Untoasted	1 slice	65	3	1	12	1.7
Toasted	1 slice	65	3	1	12	1.6
Oatmeal						
Untoasted	1 slice	73	2	1	13	1.1
Toasted	1 slice	73	2	1	13	1.1
Pita	4" pita	77	3	Tr	16	0.6
	6½" pita	165	5	1	33	1.3
Pumpernickel						
Untoasted	1 slice	80	3	1	15	2.1
Toasted	1 slice	80	3	1	15	2.1
Raisin						
Untoasted	1 slice	71	2	1	14	1.1
Toasted	1 slice	71	2	1	14	1.1
Rye						
Untoasted	1 slice	83	3	1	15	1.9
Toasted	1 slice	68	2	1	13	1.5
Rye, reduced calorie	1 slice	47	2	1	9	2.8
Wheat						
Untoasted	1 slice	65	2	1	12	1.1
Toasted	1 slice	65	2	1	12	1.2
Wheat, reduced calorie	1 slice	46	2	1	10	2.8
White						
Untoasted	1 slice	67	2	1	12	0.6
Toasted	1 slice	64	2	1	12	0.6
Soft crumbs	1 cup	120	4	2	22	1.0
White, reduced calorie	1 slice	48	2	1	10	2.2
Bread, whole wheat						
Untoasted	1 slice	69	3	1	13	1.9
Toasted	1 slice	69	3	1	13	1.9
Bread crumbs, dry, grated						
Plain, enriched	1 cup	427	14	6	78	2.6
	1 oz.	112	4	2	21	0.7
Seasoned, unenriched	1 cup	440	17	3	84	5.0

	Portion	Calories (kcal)	Protein (g)	Total Fat (g)	Carbo-hydrate (g)	Total Dietary Fiber (g)
Bread crumbs, soft (see White bread)						
Bread stuffing, prepared from dry mix	½ cup	178	3	9	22	2.9
Breakfast bar, cereal crust with fruit filling, fat free	1 bar	121	2	Tr	28	0.8
Breakfast cereals						
Hot type, cooked						
Corn (hominy) grits						
Regular or quick, enriched						
White	1 cup	145	3	Tr	31	0.5
Yellow	1 cup	145	3	Tr	31	0.5
Instant, plain	1 packet	89	2	Tr	21	1.2
Cream of Wheat						
Regular	1 cup	133	4	1	28	1.8
Quick	1 cup	129	4	Tr	27	1.2
Mix'n Eat, plain	1 packet	102	3	Tr	21	0.4
Malt-O-Meal	1 cup	122	4	Tr	26	1.0
Oatmeal						
Regular, quick or instant, plain, nonfortified	1 cup	145	6	2	25	4.0
Instant, fortified, plain	1 packet	104	4	2	18	3.0
Quaker instant						
Apples and cinnamon	1 packet	125	3	1	26	2.5
Maple and brown sugar	1 packet	153	4	2	31	2.6
Wheatena	1 cup	136	5	1	29	6.6
Ready to eat						
All-Bran	½ cup	79	4	1	23	9.7
Apple Cinnamon Cheerios	¾ cup	118	2	2	25	1.6
Apple Jacks	1 cup	116	1	Tr	27	0.6
Basic 4	1 cup	201	4	3	42	3.4
Berry Berry Kix	¾ cup	120	1	1	26	0.2
Cap'n Crunch	¾ cup	107	1	1	23	0.9

	Portion	Calories (kcal)	Protein (g)	Total Fat (g)	Carbo-hydrate (g)	Total Dietary Fiber (g)
Cap'n Crunch Crunchberries	¾ cup	104	1	1	22	0.6
Cap'n Crunch's Peanut Butter Crunch	¾ cup	112	2	2	22	0.8
Cheerios	1 cup	110	3	2	23	2.6
Chex						
Corn	1 cup	113	2	Tr	26	0.5
Honey Nut	¾ cup	117	2	1	26	0.4
Multi-Bran	1 cup	165	4	1	41	6.4
Rice	1½ cup	117	2	Tr	27	0.3
Wheat	1 cup	104	3	1	24	3.3
Cinnamon Life	1 cup	190	4	2	40	3.0
Cinnamon Toast Crunch	¾ cup	124	2	3	24	1.5
Cocoa Krispies	¾ cup	120	2	1	27	0.4
Cocoa Puffs	1 cup	119	1	1	27	0.2
Corn Flakes						
General Mills, Total	1½ cup	112	2	Tr	26	0.8
Kellogg's	1 cup	102	2	Tr	24	0.8
Corn Pops	1 cup	118	1	Tr	28	0.4
Crispix	1 cup	108	2	Tr	25	0.6
Complete Wheat Bran Flakes	¾ cup	95	3	1	23	4.6
Froot Loops	1 cup	117	1	1	26	0.6
Frosted Flakes	¾ cup	119	1	Tr	28	0.6
Frosted Mini-Wheats						
Regular	1 cup	173	5	1	42	5.5
Bite size	1 cup	187	5	1	45	5.9
Golden Grahams	¾ cup	116	2	1	26	0.9
Honey Frosted Wheaties	¾ cup	110	2	Tr	26	1.5
Honey Nut Cheerios	1 cup	115	3	1	24	1.6
Honey Nut Clusters	1 cup	213	5	3	43	4.2
Kix	1⅓ cup	114	2	1	26	0.8
Life	¾ cup	121	3	1	25	2.0
Lucky Charms	1 cup	116	2	1	25	1.2

	Portion	Calories (kcal)	Protein (g)	Total Fat (g)	Carbo-hydrate (g)	Total Dietary Fiber (g)
Nature Valley Granola	¼ cup	248	6	10	36	3.5
100% Natural Cereal						
With oats, honey, and raisins	½ cup	218	5	7	36	3.7
With raisins, low fat	½ cup	195	4	3	40	3.0
Product 19	1 cup	110	3	Tr	25	1.0
Puffed Rice	1 cup	56	1	Tr	13	0.2
Puffed Wheat	1 cup	44	2	Tr	10	0.5
Raisin Bran						
General Mills, Total	1 cup	178	4	1	43	5.0
Kellogg's	1 cup	186	6	1	47	8.2
Raisin Nut Bran	1 cup	209	5	4	41	5.1
Reese's Peanut Butter Puffs	¾ cup	129	3	3	23	0.4
Rice Krispies	1¼ cup	124	2	Tr	29	0.4
Rice Krispies Treats cereal	¾ cup	120	1	2	26	0.3
Shredded Wheat	2 biscuits	156	5	1	38	5.3
Smacks	¾ cup	103	2	1	24	0.9
Special K	1 cup	115	6	Tr	22	1.0
Quaker Toasted Oatmeal, Honey Nut	1 cup	191	5	3	39	3.3
Total, Whole Grain	¾ cup	105	3	1	24	2.6
Trix	1 cup	122	1	2	26	0.7
Wheaties	1 cup	110	3	1	24	2.1
Brownies, without icing						
Commercially prepared						
Regular, large (2¼" sq. × ⅞")	1 brownie	227	3	9	36	1.2
Fat free, 2" sq.	1 brownie	89	1	Tr	22	1.0
Prepared from dry mix, reduced calorie, 2" sq.	1 brownie	84	1	2	16	0.8
Buckwheat flour, whole groat	1 cup	402	15	4	85	12.0
Buckwheat groats, roasted (kasha), cooked	1 cup	155	6	1	33	4.5

	Portion	Calories (kcal)	Protein (g)	Total Fat (g)	Carbo-hydrate (g)	Total Dietary Fiber (g)
Bulgur						
Uncooked	1 cup	479	17	2	106	25.6
Cooked	1 cup	151	6	Tr	34	8.2
Cakes						
Cakes, prepared from dry mix						
Angelfood (¹⁄₁₂ of 10" dia.)	1 piece	129	3	Tr	29	0.1
Yellow, light, with water, egg whites, no frosting (¹⁄₁₂ of 9" dia.)	1 piece	181	3	2	37	0.6
Cakes, prepared from recipe						
Chocolate, without frosting (¹⁄₁₂ of 9" dia.)	1 piece	340	5	14	51	1.5
Gingerbread (¹⁄₉ of 8" sq.)	1 piece	263	3	12	36	0.7
Pineapple upside down (¹⁄₉ of 8" sq.)	1 piece	367	4	14	58	0.9
Shortcake, biscuit type (about 3" dia.)	1 shortcake	225	4	9	32	0.8
Sponge (¹⁄₁₂ of 16-oz. cake)	1 piece	187	5	3	36	0.4
White						
With coconut frosting (¹⁄₁₂ of 9" dia.)	1 piece	399	5	12	71	1.1
Without frosting (¹⁄₁₂ of 9" dia.)	1 piece	264	4	9	42	0.6
Cakes, commercially prepared						
Angelfood (¹⁄₁₂ of 12-oz. cake)	1 piece	72	2	Tr	16	0.4
Boston cream (¹⁄₆ of pie)	1 piece	232	2	8	39	1.3
Chocolate with chocolate frosting (¹⁄₈ of 18-oz. cake)	1 piece	235	3	10	35	1.8
Coffeecake, crumb (¹⁄₉ of 20-oz. cake)	1 piece	263	4	15	29	1.3
Fruitcake	1 piece	139	1	4	26	1.6

	Portion	Calories (kcal)	Protein (g)	Total Fat (g)	Carbo-hydrate (g)	Total Dietary Fiber (g)
Pound						
Butter (¹⁄₁₂ of 12-oz. cake)	1 piece	109	2	6	14	0.1
Fat free (3¼" × 2¾" × ⅝" slice)	1 slice	79	2	Tr	17	0.3
Snack cakes						
Chocolate, crème filled, with frosting	1 cupcake	188	2	7	30	0.4
Chocolate, with frosting, low fat	1 cupcake	131	2	2	29	1.8
Sponge, crème filled	1 cake	155	1	5	27	0.2
Sponge, individual shortcake	1 shortcake	87	2	1	18	0.2
Yellow						
With chocolate frosting	1 piece	243	2	11	35	1.2
With vanilla frosting	1 piece	239	2	9	38	0.2
Cheesecake (⅙ of 17-oz. cake)	1 piece	257	4	18	20	0.3
Cheese flavor puffs or twists	1 oz.	157	2	10	15	0.3
Chex mix	1 oz. (about ⅔ cup)	120	3	5	18	1.6
Cookies						
Butter, commercially prepared	1 cookie	23	Tr	1	3	Tr
Chocolate chip, medium (2¼"–2½" dia.)						
Commercially prepared						
Regular	1 cookie	48	1	2	7	0.3
Reduced fat	1 cookie	45	1	2	7	0.4
From refrigerated dough (spooned from roll)	1 cookie	128	1	6	18	0.4
Prepared from recipe, with margarine	1 cookie	78	1	5	9	0.4
Devil's food, commercially prepared, fat free	1 cookie	49	1	Tr	12	0.3

	Portion	Calories (kcal)	Protein (g)	Total Fat (g)	Carbo-hydrate (g)	Total Dietary Fiber (g)
Fig bar	1 cookie	56	1	1	11	0.7
Molasses						
Medium	1 cookie	65	1	2	11	0.1
Large (3½"–4" dia.)	1 cookie	138	2	4	24	0.3
Oatmeal						
Commercially prepared, with or without raisins						
Regular, large	1 cookie	113	2	5	17	0.7
Soft type	1 cookie	61	1	2	10	0.4
Fat free	1 cookie	36	1	Tr	9	0.8
Prepared from recipe, with raisins (2⅝" dia.)	1 cookie	65	1	2	10	0.5
Peanut butter						
Commercially prepared	1 cookie	72	1	4	9	0.3
Prepared from recipe, with margarine (3" dia.)	1 cookie	95	2	5	12	0.4
Sandwich type, with crème filling						
Chocolate cookie	1 cookie	47	Tr	2	7	0.3
Vanilla cookie						
Oval	1 cookie	72	1	3	11	0.2
Round	1 cookie	48	Tr	2	7	0.2
Shortbread, commercially prepared						
Plain (1⅝" sq.)	1 cookie	40	Tr	2	5	0.1
Pecan						
Regular (2" dia.)	1 cookie	76	1	5	8	0.3
Reduced fat	1 cookie	73	1	3	11	0.2
Sugar						
Commercially prepared	1 cookie	72	1	3	10	0.1
From refrigerated dough	1 cookie	73	1	3	10	0.1
Prepared from recipe, with margarine (3" dia.)	1 cookie	66	1	3	8	0.2

	Portion	Calories (kcal)	Protein (g)	Total Fat (g)	Carbo-hydrate (g)	Total Dietary Fiber (g)
Vanilla wafer, lower fat, medium size	1 cookie	18	Tr	1	3	0.1
Corn chips						
Plain	1 oz.	153	2	9	16	1.4
Barbecue flavor	1 oz.	148	2	9	16	1.5
Cornbread						
Prepared from mix, piece 3¾" × 2½" × ¾"	1 piece	188	4	6	29	1.4
Prepared from recipe, with 2% milk, piece 2½" sq. × 1½"	1 piece	173	4	5	28	1.9
Cornmeal, yellow, dry form						
Whole grain	1 cup	442	10	4	94	8.9
De-germed, enriched	1 cup	505	12	2	107	10.2
Self rising, de-germed, enriched	1 cup	490	12	2	103	9.8
Cornstarch	1 TB.	30	Tr	Tr	7	0.1
Couscous						
Uncooked	1 cup	650	22	1	134	8.7
Cooked	1 cup	176	6	Tr	36	2.2
Crackers						
Cheese, 1" sq.	10 crackers	50	1	3	6	0.2
Graham, plain 2½" sq.	2 squares	59	1	1	11	0.4
Crushed	1 cup	355	6	8	65	2.4
Melba toast, plain	4 pieces	78	2	1	15	1.3
Rye wafer, whole grain, plain	1 wafer	37	1	Tr	9	2.5
Saltine						
Square	4 crackers	52	1	1	9	0.4
Oyster type	1 cup	195	4	5	32	1.4
Sandwich type						
Wheat with cheese	1 sandwich	33	1	1	4	0.1
Cheese with peanut butter	1 sandwich	34	1	2	4	0.2
Standard snack type						
Bite size	1 cup	311	5	16	38	1.0
Round	4 crackers	60	1	3	7	0.2

	Portion	Calories (kcal)	Protein (g)	Total Fat (g)	Carbo-hydrate (g)	Total Dietary Fiber (g)
Wheat, thin square	4 crackers	38	1	2	5	0.4
Whole wheat	4 crackers	71	1	3	11	1.7
Croissant, butter	1 croissant	231	5	12	26	1.5
Croutons, seasoned	1 cup	186	4	7	25	2.0
Danish pastry, enriched						
Cheese filled	1 Danish	266	6	16	26	0.7
Fruit filled	1 Danish	263	4	13	34	1.3
Doughnuts						
Cake type	1 hole	59	1	3	7	0.2
	1 medium	198	2	11	23	0.7
Yeast leavened, glazed	1 hole	52	1	3	6	0.2
	1 medium	242	4	14	27	0.7
Eclair, prepared from recipe, 5" × 2" × 1¾"	1 eclair	262	6	16	24	0.6
English muffin, plain, enriched						
Untoasted	1 muffin	134	4	1	26	1.5
Toasted	1 muffin	133	4	1	26	1.5
French toast						
Prepared from recipe, with 2% milk, fried in margarine	1 slice	149	5	7	16	0.7
Frozen, ready to heat	1 slice	126	4	4	19	0.7
Granola bar						
Hard, plain	1 bar	134	3	6	18	1.5
Soft, uncoated						
Chocolate chip	1 bar	119	2	5	20	1.4
Raisin	1 bar	127	2	5	19	1.2
Soft, chocolate-coated, peanut butter	1 bar	144	3	9	15	0.8
Macaroni (elbows), enriched, cooked	1 cup	197	7	1	40	1.8
Matzo, plain	1 matzo	112	3	Tr	24	0.9
Muffins						
Blueberry						
Commercially prepared (2¾" dia. × 2")	1 muffin	158	3	4	27	1.5

	Portion	Calories (kcal)	Protein (g)	Total Fat (g)	Carbo-hydrate (g)	Total Dietary Fiber (g)
Prepared from mix (2¼" dia. × 1¾")	1 muffin	150	3	4	24	0.6
Prepared from recipe, with 2% milk	1 muffin	162	4	6	23	1.1
Bran with raisins, toaster type, toasted	1 muffin	106	2	3	19	2.8
Corn						
Commercially prepared (2½" dia. × 2¼")	1 muffin	174	3	5	29	1.9
Prepared from mix (2¼" dia. × 1½")	1 muffin	161	4	5	25	1.2
Oat bran, commercially prepared (2½" dia. × 2¼")	1 muffin	154	4	4	28	2.6
Noodles, chow mein, canned	1 cup	237	4	14	26	1.8
Noodles (egg noodles), enriched, cooked						
Regular	1 cup	213	8	2	40	1.8
Spinach	1 cup	211	8	3	39	3.7
Nutri-Grain Cereal Bar, fruit filled	1 bar	136	2	3	27	0.8
Oat bran						
Uncooked	1 cup	231	16	7	62	14.5
Cooked	1 cup	88	7	2	25	5.7
Oriental snack mix	1 oz. (about ¼ cup)	156	5	7	15	3.7
Pancakes, plain (4" dia.)						
Frozen, ready to heat	1 pancake	82	2	1	16	0.6
Prepared from complete mix	1 pancake	74	2	1	14	0.5
Prepared from incomplete mix, with 2% milk, egg, and oil	1 pancake	83	3	3	11	0.7
Pie crust, baked						
Standard type						
From recipe	1 pie shell	949	12	62	86	3.0
From frozen	1 pie shell	648	6	41	62	1.3
Graham cracker	1 pie shell	1,181	10	60	156	3.6

	Portion	Calories (kcal)	Protein (g)	Total Fat (g)	Carbo-hydrate (g)	Total Dietary Fiber (g)
Pies						
Commercially prepared (⅙ of 8" dia.)						
Apple	1 piece	277	2	13	40	1.9
Blueberry	1 piece	271	2	12	41	1.2
Cherry	1 piece	304	2	13	47	0.9
Chocolate crème	1 piece	344	3	22	38	2.3
Coconut custard	1 piece	270	6	14	31	1.9
Lemon meringue	1 piece	303	2	10	53	1.4
Pecan	1 piece	452	5	21	65	4.0
Pumpkin	1 piece	229	4	10	30	2.9
Prepared from recipe (⅛ of 9" dia.)						
Apple	1 piece	411	4	19	58	3.6
Blueberry	1 piece	360	4	17	49	3.6
Cherry	1 piece	486	5	22	69	3.5
Lemon meringue	1 piece	362	5	16	50	0.7
Pecan	1 piece	503	6	27	64	2.2
Pumpkin	1 piece	316	7	14	41	2.9
Fried, cherry	1 pie	404	4	21	55	3.3
Popcorn						
Air popped, unsalted	1 cup	31	1	Tr	6	1.2
Oil popped, salted	1 cup	55	1	3	6	1.1
Caramel coated						
With peanuts	1 cup	168	3	3	34	1.6
Without peanuts	1 cup	152	1	5	28	1.8
Cheese flavor	1 cup	58	1	4	6	1.1
Popcorn cake	1 cake	38	1	Tr	8	0.3
Pretzels, made with enriched flour						
Stick, 2¼" long	10 pretzels	11	Tr	Tr	2	0.1
Twisted, regular	10 pretzels	229	5	2	48	1.9
Twisted, Dutch, 2¾" × 2⅝"	1 pretzel	61	1	1	13	0.5

	Portion	Calories (kcal)	Protein (g)	Total Fat (g)	Carbo-hydrate (g)	Total Dietary Fiber (g)
Rice						
Brown, long grain, cooked	1 cup	216	5	2	45	3.5
White, long grain, enriched						
Regular						
Raw	1 cup	675	13	1	148	2.4
Cooked	1 cup	205	4	Tr	45	0.6
Instant, prepared	1 cup	162	3	Tr	35	1.0
Parboiled						
Raw	1 cup	686	13	1	151	3.1
Cooked	1 cup	200	4	Tr	43	0.7
Wild, cooked	1 cup	166	7	1	35	3.0
Rice cake, brown rice, plain	1 cake	35	1	Tr	7	0.4
Rice Krispies Treats squares	1 bar	91	1	2	18	0.1
Rolls						
Dinner	1 roll	84	2	2	14	0.8
Hamburger or hotdog	1 roll	123	4	2	22	1.2
Hard, kaiser	1 roll	167	6	2	30	1.3
Spaghetti, cooked						
Enriched	1 cup	197	7	1	40	2.4
Whole wheat	1 cup	174	7	1	37	6.3
Sweet rolls, cinnamon						
Commercial, with raisins	1 roll	223	4	10	31	1.4
Refrigerated dough, baked, with frosting	1 roll	109	2	4	17	0.6
Taco shell, baked	1 medium	62	1	3	8	1.0
Tapioca, pearl, dry	1 cup	544	Tr	Tr	135	1.4
Toaster pastries						
Brown sugar cinnamon	1 pastry	206	3	7	34	0.5
Chocolate with frosting	1 pastry	201	3	5	37	0.6
Fruit filled	1 pastry	204	2	5	37	1.1
Low fat	1 pastry	193	2	3	40	0.8

	Portion	Calories (kcal)	Protein (g)	Total Fat (g)	Carbo-hydrate (g)	Total Dietary Fiber (g)
Tortilla chips						
Plain						
Regular	1 oz.	142	2	7	18	1.8
Low fat, baked	10 chips	54	2	1	11	0.7
Nacho flavor						
Regular	1 oz.	141	2	7	18	1.5
Light, reduced fat	1 oz.	126	2	4	20	1.4
Tortillas, ready to cook (about 6" dia.)						
Corn	1 tortilla	58	1	1	12	1.4
Flour	1 tortilla	104	3	2	18	1.1
Waffles, plain						
Prepared from recipe, 7" dia.	1 waffle	218	6	11	25	0.7
Frozen, toasted, 4" dia.	1 waffle	87	2	3	13	0.8
Low fat, 4" dia.	1 waffle	83	2	1	15	0.4
Wheat flours						
All purpose, enriched						
Sifted, spooned	1 cup	419	12	1	88	3.1
Unsifted, spooned	1 cup	455	13	1	95	3.4
Bread, enriched	1 cup	495	16	2	99	3.3
Cake or pastry flour, enriched, unsifted, spooned	1 cup	496	11	1	107	2.3
Self rising, enriched, unsifted, spooned	1 cup	443	12	1	93	3.4
Whole wheat, from hard wheats, stirred, spooned	1 cup	407	16	2	87	14.6
Wheat germ, toasted, plain	1 TB.	27	2	1	3	0.9
Legumes, nuts, and seeds						
Almonds, shelled						
Sliced	1 cup	549	20	48	19	11.2
Whole	1 oz. (24 nuts)	164	6	14	6	3.3

	Portion	Calories (kcal)	Protein (g)	Total Fat (g)	Carbo-hydrate (g)	Total Dietary Fiber (g)
Beans, dry						
Cooked						
Black	1 cup	227	15	1	41	15.0
Great Northern	1 cup	209	15	1	37	12.4
Kidney, red	1 cup	225	15	1	40	13.1
Lima, large	1 cup	216	15	1	39	13.2
Pea (navy)	1 cup	258	16	1	48	11.6
Pinto	1 cup	234	14	1	44	14.7
Canned, solids and liquid						
Baked beans						
Plain or vegetarian	1 cup	236	12	1	52	12.7
With frankfurters	1 cup	368	17	17	40	17.9
With pork in tomato sauce	1 cup	248	13	3	49	12.1
With pork in sweet sauce	1 cup	281	13	4	53	13.2
Kidney, red	1 cup	218	13	1	40	16.4
Lima, large	1 cup	190	12	Tr	36	11.6
White	1 cup	307	19	1	57	12.6
Black-eyed peas, dry						
Cooked	1 cup	200	13	1	36	11.2
Canned, solids and liquid	1 cup	185	11	1	33	7.9
Brazil nuts, shelled	1 oz. (6–8 nuts)	186	4	19	4	1.5
Carob flour	1 cup	229	5	1	92	41.0
Cashews, salted						
Dry roasted	1 oz.	163	4	13	9	0.9
Oil roasted	1 cup	749	21	63	37	4.9
	1 oz. (18 nuts)	163	5	14	8	1.1
Chestnuts, European, roasted, shelled	1 cup	350	5	3	76	7.3
Chickpeas, dry						
Cooked	1 cup	269	15	4	45	12.5
Canned, solids and liquid	1 cup	286	12	3	54	10.6

	Portion	Calories (kcal)	Protein (g)	Total Fat (g)	Carbo-hydrate (g)	Total Dietary Fiber (g)
Coconut						
Raw						
Piece, about 2" × 2" × ½"	1 piece	159	1	15	7	4.1
Shredded, not packed	1 cup	283	3	27	12	7.2
Dried, sweetened, shredded	1 cup	466	3	33	44	4.2
Hazelnuts (filberts), chopped	1 cup	722	17	70	19	11.2
	1 oz.	178	4	17	5	2.7
Hummus, commercial	1 TB.	23	1	1	2	0.8
Lentils, dry, cooked	1 cup	230	18	1	40	15.6
Macadamia nuts, dry roasted, salted	1 cup 1 oz.	959	10	102	17	10.7
	(10–12 nuts)	203	2	22	4	2.3
Mixed nuts, with peanuts, salted						
Dry roasted	1 oz.	168	5	15	7	2.6
Oil roasted	1 oz.	175	5	16	6	2.6
Peanuts						
Dry roasted						
Salted	1 oz. (about 28)	166	7	14	6	2.3
Unsalted	1 cup	854	35	73	31	11.7
	1 oz. (about 28)	166	7	14	6.	2.3
Oil roasted, salted	1 cup	837	38	71	27	13.2
	1 oz.	165	7	14	5	2.6
Peanut butter						
Regular						
Smooth style	1 TB.	95	4	8	3	0.9
Chunk style	1 TB.	94	4	8	3	1.1
Reduced fat, smooth	1 TB.	94	5	6	6	0.9
Peas, split, dry, cooked	1 cup	231	16	1	41	16.3
Pecans, halves	1 cup	746	10	78	15	10.4
	1 oz. (20 halves)	196	3	20	4	2.7
Pine nuts (pignoli), shelled	1 oz.	160	7	14	4	1.3
	1 TB.	49	2	4	1	0.4

	Portion	Calories (kcal)	Protein (g)	Total Fat (g)	Carbo-hydrate (g)	Total Dietary Fiber (g)
Pistachio nuts, dry roasted, with salt, shelled	1 oz. (47 nuts)	161	6	13	8	2.9
Pumpkin and squash kernels, roasted, with salt	1 oz. (142 seeds)	148	9	12	4	1.1
Refried beans, canned	1 cup	237	14	3	39	13.4
Sesame seeds	1 TB.	47	2	4	1	0.9
Soybeans, dry, cooked	1 cup	298	29	15	17	10.3
Soy products						
Miso	1 cup	567	32	17	77	14.9
Soy milk	1 cup	81	7	5	4	3.2
Tofu						
Firm	¼ block	62	7	4	2	0.3
Soft, piece 2½" × 2¾" × 1"	1 piece	73	8	4	2	0.2
Sunflower seed kernels, dry roasted, with salt	¼ cup	186	6	16	8	2.9
	1 oz.	165	5	14	7	2.6
Tahini	1 TB.	89	3	8	3	1.4
Walnuts, English	1 cup, chopped	785	18	78	16	8.0
	1 oz. (14 halves)	185	4	18	4	1.9
Meat and meat products						
Beef, cooked						
Cuts braised, simmered, or pot roasted						
Relatively fat, such as chuck blade, piece, 2½" × 2½" × ¾"						
Lean and fat	3 oz.	293	23	22	0	0.0
Lean only	3 oz.	213	26	11	0	0.0
Relatively lean, such as bottom round, piece, 4⅛" × 2¼" × ½"						
Lean and fat	3 oz.	234	24	14	0	0.0
Lean only	3 oz.	178	27	7	0	0.0

	Portion	Calories (kcal)	Protein (g)	Total Fat (g)	Carbo-hydrate (g)	Total Dietary Fiber (g)
Ground beef, broiled						
83% lean	3 oz.	218	22	14	0	0.0
79% lean	3 oz.	231	21	16	0	0.0
73% lean	3 oz.	246	20	18	0	0.0
Liver, fried, slice, 6½" × 2⅜" × ⅜"	3 oz.	184	23	7	7	0.0
Roast, oven cooked, no liquid added						
Relatively fat, such as rib, 2 pieces, 4⅛" × 2¼" × ¼"						
Lean and fat	3 oz.	304	19	25	0	0.0
Lean only	3 oz.	195	23	11	0	0.0
Relatively lean, such as eye of round, 2 pieces, 2½" × 2½" × ⅜"						
Lean and fat	3 oz.	195	23	11	0	0.0
Lean only	3 oz.	143	25	4	0	0.0
Steak, sirloin, broiled, piece, 2½" × 2½" × ¾"						
Lean and fat	3 oz.	219	24	13	0	0.0
Lean only	3 oz.	166	26	6	0	0.0
Beef, canned, corned	3 oz.	213	23	13	0	0.0
Beef, dried, chipped	1 oz.	47	8	1	Tr	0.0
Lamb, cooked						
Chops						
Arm, braised						
Lean and fat	3 oz.	294	26	20	0	0.0
Lean only	3 oz.	237	30	12	0	0.0
Loin, broiled						
Lean and fat	3 oz.	269	21	20	0	0.0
Lean only	3 oz.	184	25	8	0	0.0
Leg, roasted, 2 pieces, 4⅛" × 2¼" × ¼"						
Lean and fat	3 oz.	219	22	14	0	0.0
Lean only	3 oz.	162	24	7	0	0.0

	Portion	Calories (kcal)	Protein (g)	Total Fat (g)	Carbo-hydrate (g)	Total Dietary Fiber (g)
Rib, roasted, 3 pieces, 2½" × 2½" × ¼"						
Lean and fat	3 oz.	305	18	25	0	0.0
Lean only	3 oz.	197	22	11	0	0.0
Pork, cured, cooked						
Bacon						
Regular	3 medium slices	109	6	9	Tr	0.0
Canadian style (6 slices per 6-oz. pkg.)	2 slices	86	11	4	1	0.0
Ham, light cure, roasted, 2 pieces, 4⅛" × 2¼" × ¼"						
Lean and fat	3 oz.	207	18	14	0	0.0
Lean only	3 oz.	133	21	5	0	0.0
Ham, canned, roasted, 2 pieces, 4⅛" × 2¼" × ¼"	3 oz.	142	18	7	Tr	0.0
Pork, fresh, cooked						
Chop, loin (cut 3 per lb. with bone)						
Broiled						
Lean and fat	3 oz.	204	24	11	0	0.0
Lean only	3 oz.	172	26	7	0	0.0
Pan fried						
Lean and fat	3 oz.	235	25	14	0	0.0
Lean only	3 oz.	197	27	9	0	0.0
Ham (leg), roasted, piece, 2½" × 2½" × ¼"						
Lean and fat	3 oz.	232	23	15	0	0.0
Lean only	3 oz.	179	25	8	0	0.0
Rib roast, piece, 2½" × 2½" × ¾"						
Lean and fat	3 oz.	217	23	13	0	0.0
Lean only	3 oz.	190	24	9	0	0.0

	Portion	Calories (kcal)	Protein (g)	Total Fat (g)	Carbo-hydrate (g)	Total Dietary Fiber (g)
Ribs, lean and fat, cooked						
Backribs, roasted	3 oz.	315	21	25	0	0.0
Country style, braised	3 oz.	252	20	18	0	0.0
Spareribs, braised	3 oz.	337	25	26	0	0.0
Shoulder cut, braised, 3 pieces, 2½" × 2½" × ¼"						
Lean and fat	3 oz.	280	24	20	0	0.0
Lean only	3 oz.	211	27	10	0	0.0
Sausages and luncheon meats						
Bologna, beef and pork (8 slices per 8-oz. pkg.)	2 slices	180	7	16	2	0.0
Braunschweiger (6 slices per 6-oz. pkg.)	2 slices	205	8	18	2	0.0
Brown and serve, cooked, link, 4" × ⅞" raw	2 links	103	4	9	1	0.0
Canned, minced luncheon meat						
Pork, ham, and chicken, reduced sodium (7 slices per 7-oz. can)	2 slices	172	7	15	1	0.0
Pork with ham (12 slices per 12-oz. can)	2 slices	188	8	17	1	0.0
Pork and chicken (12 slices per 12-oz. can)	2 slices	117	9	8	1	0.0
Chopped ham (8 slices per 6-oz. pkg.)	2 slices	48	4	4	0	0.0
Cooked ham (8 slices per 8-oz. pkg.)						
Regular	2 slices	104	10	6	2	0.0
Extra lean	2 slices	75	11	3	1	0.0
Frankfurter (10 per 1-lb. pkg.), heated						
Beef and pork	1 frank	144	5	13	1	0.0
Beef	1 frank	142	5	13	1	0.0
Pork sausage, fresh, cooked						
Link (4" × ⅞" raw)	2 links	96	5	8	Tr	0.0
Patty (3⅞" × ¼" raw)	1 patty	100	5	8	Tr	0.0

	Portion	Calories (kcal)	Protein (g)	Total Fat (g)	Carbo-hydrate (g)	Total Dietary Fiber (g)
Salami, beef and pork						
Cooked type (8 slices per 8-oz. pkg.)	2 slices	143	8	11	1	0.0
Dry type, slice, 3⅛" × ¹⁄₁₆"	2 slices	84	5	7	1	0.0
Sandwich spread (pork, beef)	1 TB.	35	1	3	2	Tr
Vienna sausage (7 per 4-oz. can)	1 sausage	45	2	4	Tr	0.0
Veal, lean and fat, cooked						
Cutlet, braised, 4⅛" × 2¼" × ½"	3 oz.	179	31	5	0	0.0
Rib, roasted, 2 pieces, 4⅛" × 2¼" × ¼"	3 oz.	194	20	12	0	0.0

Mixed dishes and fast foods

	Portion	Calories (kcal)	Protein (g)	Total Fat (g)	Carbo-hydrate (g)	Total Dietary Fiber (g)
Mixed dishes						
Beef macaroni, frozen, Healthy Choice	1 package	211	14	2	33	4.6
Beef stew, canned	1 cup	218	11	12	16	3.5
Chicken pot pie, frozen	1 small pie	484	13	29	43	1.7
Chili con carne with beans, canned	1 cup	255	20	8	24	8.2
Macaroni and cheese, canned, made with corn oil	1 cup	199	8	6	29	3.0
Meatless burger crumbles, Morningstar Farms	1 cup	231	22	13	7	5.1
Meatless burger patty, frozen, Morningstar Farms	1 patty	91	14	1	8	4.3
Pasta with meatballs in tomato sauce, canned	1 cup	260	11	10	31	6.8
Spaghetti bolognese (meat sauce), frozen, Healthy Choice	1 package	255	14	3	43	5.1
Spaghetti in tomato sauce with cheese, canned	1 cup	192	6	2	39	7.8
Spinach souffle, home-prepared	1 cup	219	11	18	3	NA

	Portion	Calories (kcal)	Protein (g)	Total Fat (g)	Carbo-hydrate (g)	Total Dietary Fiber (g)
Tortellini, pasta with cheese filling, frozen	¾ cup (yields 1 cup cooked)	249	11	6	38	1.5
Fast foods						
Breakfast items						
Biscuit with egg and sausage	1 biscuit	581	19	39	41	0.9
Croissant with egg, cheese, bacon	1 croissant	413	16	28	24	NA
Danish pastry						
Cheese filled	1 pastry	353	6	25	29	NA
Fruit filled	1 pastry	335	5	16	45	NA
English muffin with egg, cheese, Canadian bacon	1 muffin	289	17	13	27	1.5
French toast with butter	2 slices	356	10	19	36	NA
French toast sticks	5 sticks	513	8	29	58	2.7
Hashed brown potatoes	½ cup	151	2	9	16	NA
Pancakes with butter, syrup	2 pancakes	520	8	14	91	NA
Burrito						
With beans and cheese	1 burrito	189	8	6	27	NA
With beans and meat	1 burrito	255	11	9	33	NA
Cheeseburger						
Regular size, with condiments						
Double patty with mayo-type dressing, vegetables	1 sandwich	417	21	21	35	NA
Single patty	1 sandwich	295	16	14	27	NA
Regular size, plain						
Double patty	1 sandwich	457	28	28	22	NA
Double patty with 3-piece bun	1 sandwich	461	22	22	44	NA
Single patty	1 sandwich	319	15	15	32	NA
Large, with condiments						
Single patty with mayo-type dressing, vegetables	1 sandwich	563	28	33	38	NA
Single patty with bacon	1 sandwich	608	32	37	37	NA

	Portion	Calories (kcal)	Protein (g)	Total Fat (g)	Carbo-hydrate (g)	Total Dietary Fiber (g)
Chicken fillet (breaded and fried) sandwich, plain	1 sandwich	515	24	29	39	NA
Chicken, fried (See Poultry and poultry products)						
Chicken pieces, boneless, breaded and fried, plain	6 pieces	319	18	21	15	0.0
Chili con carne	1 cup	256	25	8	22	NA
Chimichanga with beef	1 chimi-changa	425	20	20	43	NA
Coleslaw	¾ cup	147	1	11	13	NA
Desserts						
Ice milk, soft, vanilla, in cone	1 cone	164	4	6	24	0.1
Pie, fried, with fruit filling (5" × 3¾")	1 pie	404	4	21	55	3.3
Sundae, hot fudge	1 sundae	284	6	9	48	0.0
Enchilada with cheese	1 enchilada	319	10	19	29	NA
Fish sandwich, with tartar sauce and cheese	1 sandwich	523	21	29	48	NA
French fries	1 small	291	4	16	34	3.0
	1 medium	458	6	25	53	4.7
	1 large	578	7	31	67	5.9
Frijoles (refried beans, chili sauce, cheese)	1 cup	225	11	8	29	NA
Hamburger						
Regular size, with condiments						
Double patty	1 sandwich	576	32	32	39	NA
Single patty	1 sandwich	272	12	10	34	2.3
Large, with condiments, mayo-type dressing, and vegetables						
Double patty	1 sandwich	540	34	27	40	NA
Single patty	1 sandwich	512	26	27	40	NA
Hot dog						
Plain	1 sandwich	242	10	15	18	NA
With chili	1 sandwich	296	14	13	31	NA
With corn flour coating (corndog)	1 corndog	460	17	19	56	NA

	Portion	Calories (kcal)	Protein (g)	Total Fat (g)	Carbo-hydrate (g)	Total Dietary Fiber (g)
Hush puppies	5 pieces	257	5	12	35	NA
Mashed potatoes	⅓ cup	66	2	1	13	NA
Nachos, with cheese sauce	6–8 nachos	346	9	19	36	NA
Onion rings, breaded and fried	8–9 rings	276	4	16	31	NA
Pizza (slice = ⅛ of 12" pizza)						
Cheese	1 slice	140	8	3	21	NA
Meat and vegetables	1 slice	184	13	5	21	NA
Pepperoni	1 slice	181	10	7	20	NA
Roast beef sandwich, plain	1 sandwich	346	22	14	33	NA
Salad, tossed, with chicken, no dressing	1 ½ cups	105	17	2	4	NA
Salad, tossed, with egg, cheese, no dressing	1 ½ cups	102	9	6	5	NA
Shake						
Chocolate	16 fl. oz.	423	11	12	68	2.7
Vanilla	16 fl. oz.	370	12	10	60	1.3
Shrimp, breaded and fried	6–8 shrimp	454	19	25	40	NA
Submarine sandwich (6" long), with oil and vinegar						
Cold cuts (with lettuce, cheese, salami, ham, tomato, onion)	1 sandwich	456	22	19	51	NA
Roast beef (with tomato, lettuce, mayo)	1 sandwich	410	29	13	44	NA
Tuna salad (with mayo, lettuce)	1 sandwich	584	30	28	55	NA
Taco, beef	1 small	369	21	21	27	NA
	1 large	568	32	32	41	NA
Taco salad (with ground beef, cheese, taco shell)	1 ½ cups	279	13	15	24	NA
Tostada (with cheese, tomato, lettuce)						
With beans and beef	1 tostada	333	16	17	30	NA
With guacamole	1 tostada	181	6	12	16	NA

	Portion	Calories (kcal)	Protein (g)	Total Fat (g)	Carbo-hydrate (g)	Total Dietary Fiber (g)
		Poultry and poultry products				
Chicken						
Fried in vegetable shortening, meat with skin						
Batter dipped						
Breast, ½ breast (5.6 oz. with bones)	½ breast	364	35	18	13	0.4
Drumstick (3.4 oz. with bones)	1 drumstick	193	16	11	6	0.2
Thigh	1 thigh	238	19	14	8	0.3
Wing	1 wing	159	10	11	5	0.1
Flour coated						
Breast, ½ breast (4.2 oz. with bones)	½ breast	218	31	9	2	0.1
Drumstick (2.6 oz. with bones)	1 drumstick	120	13	7	1	Tr
Fried, meat only						
Dark meat	3 oz.	203	25	10	2	0.0
Light meat	3 oz.	163	28	5	Tr	0.0
Roasted, meat only						
Breast, ½ breast (4.2 oz. with bone and skin)	½ breast	142	27	3	0	0.0
Drumstick (2.9 oz. with bone and skin)	1 drumstick	76	12	2	0	0.0
Thigh	1 thigh	109	13	6	0	0.0
Stewed, meat only, light and dark meat, chopped or diced	1 cup	332	43	17	0	0.0
Chicken giblets, simmered, chopped	1 cup	228	37	7	1	0.0
Chicken liver, simmered	1 liver	31	5	1	Tr	0.0
Chicken neck, meat only, simmered	1 neck	32	4	1	0	0.0
Duck, roasted, flesh only	½ duck	444	52	25	0	0.0

	Portion	Calories (kcal)	Protein (g)	Total Fat (g)	Carbo-hydrate (g)	Total Dietary Fiber (g)
Turkey						
Roasted, meat only						
Dark meat	3 oz.	159	24	6	0	0.0
Light meat	3 oz.	133	25	3	0	0.0
Light and dark meat, chopped or diced	1 cup	238	41	7	0	0.0
Ground, cooked						
Patty, from 4 oz. raw	1 patty	193	22	11	0	0.0
Crumbled	1 cup	298	35	17	0	0.0
Turkey giblets, simmered, chopped	1 cup	242	39	7	3	0.0
Turkey neck, meat only, simmered	1 neck	274	41	11	0	0.0
Poultry food products						
Chicken						
Canned, boneless	5 oz.	234	31	11	0	0.0
Frankfurter (10 per 1-lb. pkg.)	1 frank	116	6	9	3	0.0
Roll, light meat (6 slices per 6-oz. pkg.)	2 slices	90	11	4	1	0.0
Turkey						
Gravy and turkey, frozen	5-oz. package	95	8	4	7	0.0
Patties, breaded or battered, fried (2.25 oz.)	1 patty	181	9	12	10	0.3
Roast, boneless, frozen, seasoned, light and dark meat, cooked	3 oz.	132	18	5	3	0.0

Soups, sauces, and gravies

	Portion	Calories (kcal)	Protein (g)	Total Fat (g)	Carbo-hydrate (g)	Total Dietary Fiber (g)
Soups						
Canned, condensed						
Prepared with equal volume of whole milk						
Clam chowder, New England	1 cup	164	9	7	17	1.5
Cream of chicken	1 cup	191	7	11	15	0.2
Cream of mushroom	1 cup	203	6	14	15	0.5
Tomato	1 cup	161	6	6	22	2.7

	Portion	Calories (kcal)	Protein (g)	Total Fat (g)	Carbo-hydrate (g)	Total Dietary Fiber (g)
Prepared with equal volume of water						
Bean with pork	1 cup	172	8	6	23	8.6
Beef broth, bouillon, consommé	1 cup	29	5	0	2	0.0
Beef noodle	1 cup	83	5	3	9	0.7
Chicken noodle	1 cup	75	4	2	9	0.7
Chicken and rice	1 cup	60	4	2	7	0.7
Clam chowder, Manhattan	1 cup	78	2	2	12	1.5
Cream of chicken	1 cup	117	3	7	9	0.2
Cream of mushroom	1 cup	129	2	9	9	0.5
Minestrone	1 cup	82	4	3	11	1.0
Pea, green	1 cup	165	9	3	27	2.8
Tomato	1 cup	85	2	2	17	0.5
Vegetable beef	1 cup	78	6	2	10	0.5
Vegetarian vegetable	1 cup	72	2	2	12	0.5
Canned, ready to serve, chunky						
Bean with ham	1 cup	231	13	9	27	11.2
Chicken noodle	1 cup	175	13	6	17	3.8
Chicken and vegetable	1 cup	166	12	5	19	NA
Vegetable	1 cup	122	4	4	19	1.2
Canned, ready to serve, low fat, reduced sodium						
Chicken broth	1 cup	17	3	0	1	0.0
Chicken noodle	1 cup	76	6	2	9	1.2
Chicken and rice	1 cup	116	7	3	14	0.7
Chicken and rice with vegetables	1 cup	88	6	1	12	0.7
Clam chowder, New England	1 cup	117	5	2	20	1.2
Lentil	1 cup	126	8	2	20	5.6
Minestrone	1 cup	123	5	3	20	1.2
Vegetable	1 cup	81	4	1	13	1.4

	Portion	Calories (kcal)	Protein (g)	Total Fat (g)	Carbo-hydrate (g)	Total Dietary Fiber (g)
Dehydrated						
Unprepared						
Beef bouillon	1 packet	14	1	1	1	0.0
Onion	1 packet	115	5	2	21	4.1
Prepared with water						
Chicken noodle	1 cup	58	2	1	9	0.3
Onion	1 cup	27	1	1	5	1.0
Home prepared, stock						
Beef	1 cup	31	5	Tr	3	0.0
Chicken	1 cup	86	6	3	8	0.0
Fish	1 cup	40	5	2	0	0.0
Sauces						
Home recipe						
Cheese	1 cup	479	25	36	13	0.2
White, medium, made with whole milk	1 cup	368	10	27	23	0.5
Ready to serve						
Barbecue	1 TB.	12	Tr	Tr	2	0.2
Cheese	¼ cup	110	4	8	4	0.3
Hoisin	1 TB.	35	1	1	7	0.4
Nacho cheese	¼ cup	119	5	10	3	0.5
Pepper or hot	1 tsp.	1	Tr	Tr	Tr	0.1
Salsa	1 TB.	4	Tr	Tr	1	0.3
Soy	1 TB.	9	1	Tr	1	0.1
Spaghetti/marinara/pasta	1 cup	143	4	5	21	4.0
Teriyaki	1 TB.	15	1	0	3	Tr
Tomato chili	¼ cup	71	2	Tr	17	4.0
Worcestershire	1 TB.	11	0	0	3	0.0
Gravies, canned						
Beef	¼ cup	31	2	1	3	0.2
Chicken	¼ cup	47	1	3	3	0.2
Country sausage	¼ cup	96	3	8	4	0.4
Mushroom	¼ cup	30	1	2	3	0.2
Turkey	¼ cup	31	2	1	3	0.2

	Portion	Calories (kcal)	Protein (g)	Total Fat (g)	Carbo-hydrate (g)	Total Dietary Fiber (g)
		Sugars and sweets				
Candy						
Butterfinger (Nestlé)	1 fun size bar	34	1	1	5	0.2
Caramel, plain	1 piece	39	Tr	1	8	0.1
Chocolate flavored roll	1 piece	25	Tr	Tr	6	Tr
Carob	1 oz.	153	2	9	16	1.1
Chocolate, milk						
Plain	1 bar (1.55 oz.)	226	3	14	26	1.5
With almonds	1 bar (1.45 oz.)	216	4	14	22	2.5
With peanuts, Mr. Goodbar (Hershey's)	1 bar (1.75 oz.)	267	5	17	25	1.7
With rice cereal, Nestlé Crunch	1 bar (1.55 oz.)	230	3	12	29	1.1
Chocolate chips						
Milk	1 cup	862	12	52	99	5.7
Semisweet	1 cup	805	7	50	106	9.9
White	1 cup	916	10	55	101	0.0
Chocolate coated peanuts	10 pieces	208	5	13	20	1.9
Chocolate coated raisins	10 pieces	39	Tr	1	7	0.4
Fruit leather, pieces	1 oz.	97	Tr	2	22	1.0
Fruit leather, rolls	1 large	74	Tr	1	18	0.8
	1 small	49	Tr	Tr	12	0.5
Fudge, prepared from recipe						
Chocolate						
Plain	1 piece	65	Tr	1	14	0.1
With nuts	1 piece	81	1	3	14	0.2
Vanilla						
Plain	1 piece	59	Tr	1	13	0.0
With nuts	1 piece	62	Tr	2	11	0.1
Gumdrops/ gummy candies						
Gumdrops (¾" dia.)	1 cup	703	0	0	180	0.0
	1 medium	16	0	0	4	0.0

	Portion	Calories (kcal)	Protein (g)	Total Fat (g)	Carbo-hydrate (g)	Total Dietary Fiber (g)
Gummy bears	10 bears	85	0	0	22	0.0
Gummy worms	10 worms	286	0	0	73	0.0
Hard candy	1 piece	24	0	Tr	6	0.0
	1 small piece	12	0	Tr	3	0.0
Jelly beans	10 large	104	0	Tr	26	0.0
	10 small	40	0	Tr	10	0.0
Kit Kat (Hershey's)	1 bar (1.5 oz.)	216	3	11	27	0.8
Marshmallows						
Miniature	1 cup	159	1	Tr	41	0.1
Regular	1 regular	23	Tr	Tr	6	Tr
M&M's (M&M Mars)						
Peanut	¼ cup	222	4	11	26	1.5
	10 pieces	103	2	5	12	0.7
Plain	¼ cup	256	2	11	37	1.3
	10 pieces	34	Tr	1	5	0.2
Milky Way	1 fun size bar	76	1	3	13	0.3
(M&M Mars)	1 bar (2.15 oz.)	258	3	10	44	1.0
Reese's Peanut Butter Cup	1 miniature cup	38	1	2	4	0.2
(Hershey's)	1 package (contains 2)	243	5	14	25	1.4
Snickers bar (M&M Mars)	1 fun size bar	72	1	4	9	0.4
	1 king size bar (4 oz.)	541	9	28	67	2.8
	1 bar (2 oz.)	273	5	14	34	1.4
Special Dark sweet chocolate (Hershey's)	1 miniature	46	Tr	3	5	0.4
Starburst fruit chews	1 piece	20	Tr	Tr	4	0.0
(M&M Mars)	1 package (2.07 oz.)	234	Tr	5	50	0.0
Frosting, ready to eat						
Chocolate	1/12 package	151	Tr	7	24	0.2
Vanilla	1/12 package	159	Tr	6	26	Tr
Frozen desserts (nondairy)						
Fruit and juice bar	1 bar (2.5 fl. oz.)	63	1	Tr	16	0.0

	Portion	Calories (kcal)	Protein (g)	Total Fat (g)	Carbo-hydrate (g)	Total Dietary Fiber (g)
Ice pop	1 bar (2 fl. oz.)	42	0	0	11	0.0
Italian ices	½ cup	61	Tr	Tr	16	0.0
Fruit butter, apple	1 TB.	29	Tr	0	7	0.3
Gelatin dessert, prepared with gelatin dessert powder and water						
Regular	½ cup	80	2	0	19	0.0
Reduced calorie (with aspartame)	½ cup	8	1	0	1	0.0
Honey, strained or extracted	1 TB.	64	Tr	0	17	Tr
	1 cup	1,031	1	0	279	0.7
Jams and preserves	1 TB.	56	Tr	Tr	14	0.2
	1 packet (0.5 oz.)	39	Tr	Tr	10	0.2
Jellies	1 TB.	54	Tr	Tr	13	0.2
	1 packet (0.5 oz.)	40	Tr	Tr	10	0.1
Puddings						
Prepared with dry mix and 2% milk						
Chocolate						
Instant	½ cup	150	5	3	28	0.6
Regular (cooked)	½cup	151	5	3	28	0.4
Vanilla						
Instant	½ cup	148	4	2	28	0.0
Regular (cooked)	½ cup	141	4	2	26	0.0
Ready to eat						
Regular						
Chocolate	4 oz.	150	3	5	26	1.1
Rice	4 oz.	184	2	8	25	0.1
Tapioca	4 oz.	134	2	4	22	0.1
Vanilla	4 oz.	147	3	4	25	0.1
Fat free						
Chocolate	4 oz.	107	3	Tr	23	0.9
Tapioca	4 oz.	98	2	Tr	23	0.1
Vanilla	4 oz.	105	2	Tr	24	0.1

	Portion	Calories (kcal)	Protein (g)	Total Fat (g)	Carbo- hydrate (g)	Total Dietary Fiber (g)
Sugar						
Brown						
Packed	1 cup	827	0	0	214	0.0
Unpacked	1 cup	545	0	0	141	0.0
	1 TB.	34	0	0	9	0.0
White						
Granulated	1 packet	23	0	0	6	0.0
	1 tsp	16	0	0	4	0.0
	1 cup	774	0	0	200	0.0
Powdered, unsifted	1 TB.	31	0	Tr	8	0.0
	1 cup	467	0	Tr	119	0.0
Syrup						
Chocolate flavored syrup or topping						
Thin type	1 TB.	53	Tr	Tr	12	0.3
Fudge type	1 TB.	67	1	2	12	0.5
Corn, light	1 TB.	56	0	0	15	0.0
Maple	1 TB.	52	0	Tr	13	0.0
Molasses, blackstrap	1 TB.	47	0	0	12	0.0
	1 cup	771	0	0	199	0.0
Table blend, pancake						
Regular	1 TB.	57	0	0	15	0.0
Reduced calorie	1 TB.	25	0	0	7	0.0
Vegetables and vegetable products						
Alfalfa sprouts, raw	1 cup	10	1	Tr	1	0.8
Artichokes, globe or French, cooked, drained	1 cup	84	6	Tr	19	9.1
	1 medium	60	4	Tr	13	6.5
Asparagus, green						
Cooked, drained						
From raw	1 cup	43	5	1	8	2.9
	4 spears	14	2	Tr	3	1.0
From frozen	1 cup	50	5	1	9	2.9
	4 spears	17	2	Tr	3	1.0
Canned, spears, about 5" long, drained	1 cup	46	5	2	6	3.9
	4 spears	14	2	Tr	2	1.2

	Portion	Calories (kcal)	Protein (g)	Total Fat (g)	Carbo-hydrate (g)	Total Dietary Fiber (g)
Bamboo shoots, canned, drained	1 cup	25	2	1	4	1.8
Beans						
Lima, immature seeds, frozen, cooked, drained						
Ford hooks	1 cup	170	10	1	32	9.9
Baby limas	1 cup	189	12	1	35	10.8
Snap, cut						
Cooked, drained						
From raw						
Green	1 cup	44	2	Tr	10	4.0
Yellow	1 cup	44	2	Tr	10	4.1
From frozen						
Green	1 cup	38	2	Tr	9	4.1
Yellow	1 cup	38	2	Tr	9	4.1
Canned, drained						
Green	1 cup	27	2	Tr	6	2.6
Yellow	1 cup	27	2	Tr	6	1.8
Beans, dry (see Legumes, nuts, and seeds)						
Bean sprouts (mung)						
Raw	1 cup	31	3	Tr	6	1.9
Cooked, drained	1 cup	26	3	Tr	5	1.5
Beets						
Cooked, drained						
Slices	1 cup	75	3	Tr	17	3.4
Whole beet, 2" dia.	1 beet	22	1	Tr	5	1.0
Canned, drained						
Slices	1 cup	53	2	Tr	12	2.9
Whole beet	1 beet	7	Tr	Tr	2	0.4
Beet greens, leaves and stems, cooked, drained, 1" pieces	1 cup	39	4	Tr	8	4.2
Black-eyed peas, immature seeds, cooked, drained						
From raw	1 cup	160	5	1	34	8.3
From frozen	1 cup	224	14	1	40	10.9

	Portion	Calories (kcal)	Protein (g)	Total Fat (g)	Carbo-hydrate (g)	Total Dietary Fiber (g)
Broccoli						
Raw						
Chopped or diced	1 cup	25	3	Tr	5	2.6
Spear, about 5" long	1 spear	9	1	Tr	2	0.9
Flower cluster	1 floweret	3	Tr	Tr	1	0.3
Cooked, drained						
From raw						
Chopped	1 cup	44	5	1	8	4.5
Spear, about 5" long	1 spear	10	1	Tr	2	1.1
From frozen, chopped	1 cup	52	6	Tr	10	5.5
Brussels sprouts, cooked, drained						
From raw	1 cup	61	4	1	14	4.1
From frozen	1 cup	65	6	1	13	6.4
Cabbage, common varieties, shredded						
Raw	1 cup	18	1	Tr	4	1.6
Cooked, drained	1 cup	33	2	1	7	3.5
Cabbage, Chinese, shredded, cooked, drained						
Pak choi or bok choy	1 cup	20	3	Tr	3	2.7
Pe tsai	1 cup	17	2	Tr	3	3.2
Cabbage, red, raw, shredded	1 cup	19	1	Tr	4	1.4
Cabbage, savoy, raw, shredded	1 cup	19	1	Tr	4	2.2
Carrot juice, canned	1 cup	94	2	Tr	22	1.9
Carrots						
Raw						
Whole, 7½" long	1 carrot	31	1	Tr	7	2.2
Grated	1 cup	47	1	Tr	11	3.3
Baby	1 medium	4	Tr	Tr	1	0.2
Cooked, sliced, drained						
From raw	1 cup	70	2	Tr	16	5.1
From frozen	1 cup	53	2	Tr	12	5.1
Canned, sliced, drained	1 cup	37	1	Tr	8	2.2

	Portion	Calories (kcal)	Protein (g)	Total Fat (g)	Carbo-hydrate (g)	Total Dietary Fiber (g)
Cauliflower						
Raw	1 floweret	3	Tr	Tr	1	0.3
	1 cup	25	2	Tr	5	2.5
Cooked, drained, 1" pieces						
From raw	1 cup	29	2	1	5	3.3
	3 flowerets	12	1	Tr	2	1.5
From frozen	1 cup	34	3	Tr	7	4.9
Celery						
Raw						
Stalk, 7½–8" long	1 stalk	6	Tr	Tr	1	0.7
Pieces, diced	1 cup	19	1	Tr	4	2.0
Cooked, drained						
Stalk, medium	1 stalk	7	Tr	Tr	2	0.6
Pieces, diced	1 cup	27	1	Tr	6	2.4
Chives, raw, chopped	1 TB.	1	Tr	Tr	Tr	0.1
Cilantro, raw	1 tsp.	Tr	Tr	Tr	Tr	Tr
Coleslaw, home prepared	1 cup	83	2	3	15	1.8
Collards, cooked, drained, chopped						
From raw	1 cup	49	4	1	9	5.3
From frozen	1 cup	61	5	1	12	4.8
Corn, sweet, yellow						
Cooked, drained						
From raw, kernels on cob	1 ear	83	3	1	19	2.2
From frozen						
Kernels on cob	1 ear	59	2	Tr	14	1.8
Kernels	1 cup	131	5	1	32	3.9
Canned						
Cream style	1 cup	184	4	1	46	3.1
Whole kernel, vacuum pack	1 cup	166	5	1	41	4.2
Corn, sweet, white, cooked, drained*	1 ear	83	3	1	19	2.1

White varieties contain only a trace amount of vitamin A; other nutrients are the same.

	Portion	Calories (kcal)	Protein (g)	Total Fat (g)	Carbohydrate (g)	Total Dietary Fiber (g)
Cucumber						
Peeled						
Sliced	1 cup	14	1	Tr	3	0.8
Whole, 8¼" long	1 large	34	2	Tr	7	2.0
Unpeeled						
Sliced	1 cup	14	1	Tr	3	0.8
Whole, 8¼" long	1 large	39	2	Tr	8	2.4
Dandelion greens, cooked, drained	1 cup	35	2	1	7	3.0
Dill weed, raw	5 sprigs	Tr	Tr	Tr	Tr	Tr
Eggplant, cooked, drained	1 cup	28	1	Tr	7	2.5
Endive, curly (including escarole), raw, small pieces	1 cup	9	1	Tr	2	1.6
Garlic, raw	1 clove	4	Tr	Tr	1	0.1
Hearts of palm, canned	1 piece	9	1	Tr	2	0.8
Jerusalem artichoke, raw, sliced	1 cup	114	3	Tr	26	2.4
Kale, cooked, drained, chopped						
From raw	1 cup	36	2	1	7	2.6
From frozen	1 cup	39	4	1	7	2.6
Kohlrabi, cooked, drained, slices	1 cup	48	3	Tr	11	1.8
Leeks, bulb and lower leaf portion, chopped or diced, cooked, drained	1 cup	32	1	Tr	8	1.0
Lettuce, raw						
Butterhead, as Boston types						
Leaf	1 medium leaf	1	Tr	Tr	Tr	0.1
Head, 5" dia.	1 head	21	2	Tr	4	1.6
Crisphead, as iceberg						
Leaf	1 medium	1	Tr	Tr	Tr	0.1
Head, 6" dia.	1 head	65	5	1	11	7.5
Pieces, shredded or chopped	1 cup	7	1	Tr	1	0.8

	Portion	Calories (kcal)	Protein (g)	Total Fat (g)	Carbo-hydrate (g)	Total Dietary Fiber (g)
Looseleaf						
Leaf	1 leaf	2	Tr	Tr	Tr	0.2
Pieces, shredded	1 cup	10	1	Tr	2	1.1
Romaine innerleaf	1 leaf	1	Tr	Tr	Tr	0.2
Pieces, shredded	1 cup	8	1	Tr	1	1.0
Mushrooms						
Raw, pieces or slices	1 cup	18	2	Tr	3	0.8
Cooked, drained, pieces	1 cup	42	3	1	8	3.4
Canned, drained, pieces	1 cup	37	3	Tr	8	3.7
Mushrooms, shiitake						
Cooked pieces	1 cup	80	2	Tr	21	3.0
Dried	1 mushroom	11	Tr	Tr	3	0.4
Mustard greens, cooked, drained	1 cup	21	3	Tr	3	2.8
Okra, sliced, cooked, drained						
From raw	1 cup	51	3	Tr	12	4.0
From frozen	1 cup	52	4	1	11	5.2
Onions						
Raw						
Chopped	1 cup	61	2	Tr	14	2.9
Whole, medium, 2½" dia.	1 whole	42	1	Tr	9	2.0
Slice, ⅛" thick	1 slice	5	Tr	Tr	1	0.3
Cooked (whole or sliced), drained	1 cup	92	3	Tr	21	2.9
	1 medium	41	1	Tr	10	1.3
Dehydrated flakes	1 TB.	17	Tr	Tr	4	0.5
Onions, spring, raw, top and bulb						
Chopped	1 cup	32	2	Tr	7	2.6
Whole, medium, 4⅛" long	1 whole	5	Tr	Tr	1	0.4
Onion rings, 2"–3" dia., breaded, pan fried, frozen, oven heated	10 rings	244	3	16	23	0.8

	Portion	Calories (kcal)	Protein (g)	Total Fat (g)	Carbo-hydrate (g)	Total Dietary Fiber (g)
Parsley, raw	10 sprigs	4	Tr	Tr	1	0.3
Parsnips, sliced, cooked, drained	1 cup	126	2	Tr	30	6.2
Peas, edible pod, cooked, drained						
From raw	1 cup	67	5	Tr	11	4.5
From frozen	1 cup	83	6	1	14	5.0
Peas, green						
Canned, drained	1 cup	117	8	1	21	7.0
Frozen, boiled, drained	1 cup	125	8	Tr	23	8.8
Peppers						
Hot chili, raw						
Green	1 pepper	18	1	Tr	4	0.7
Red	1 pepper	18	1	Tr	4	0.7
Jalapeño, canned, sliced, solids and liquids	¼ cup	7	Tr	Tr	1	0.7
Sweet (2¾" long, 2½" dia.)						
Raw						
Green						
Chopped	1 cup	40	1	Tr	10	2.7
Ring (¼" thick)	1 ring	3	Tr	Tr	1	0.2
Whole (2¾" × 2½")	1 pepper	32	1	Tr	8	2.1
Red						
Chopped	1 cup	40	1	Tr	10	3.0
Whole (2¾" × 2½")	1 pepper	32	1	Tr	8	2.4
Cooked, drained, chopped						
Green	1 cup	38	1	Tr	9	1.6
Red	1 cup	38	1	Tr	9	1.6
Pimento, canned	1 TB.	3	Tr	Tr	1	0.2

	Portion	Calories (kcal)	Protein (g)	Total Fat (g)	Carbo-hydrate (g)	Total Dietary Fiber (g)
Potatoes						
Baked (2⅓" × 4¾")						
With skin	1 potato	220	5	Tr	51	4.8
Flesh only	1 potato	145	3	Tr	34	2.3
Skin only	1 skin	115	2	Tr	27	4.6
Boiled (2½" dia.)						
Peeled after boiling	1 potato	118	3	Tr	27	2.4
Peeled before boiling	1 potato	116	2	Tr	27	2.4
	1 cup	134	3	Tr	31	2.8
Potato products, prepared						
Au gratin						
From dry mix, with whole milk, butter	1 cup	228	6	10	31	2.2
From home recipe, with butter	1 cup	323	12	19	28	4.4
French fried, frozen, oven heated	10 strips	100	2	4	16	1.6
Hashed brown						
From frozen (about 3" × 1½" × ½")	1 patty	63	1	3	8	0.6
From home recipe	1 cup	326	4	22	33	3.1
Mashed						
From dehydrated flakes (without milk); whole milk, butter, and salt added	1 cup	237	4	12	32	4.8
From home recipe						
With whole milk	1 cup	162	4	1	37	4.2
With whole milk and margarine	1 cup	223	4	9	35	4.2
Potato pancakes, home prepared	1 pancake	207	5	12	22	1.5
Potato puffs, from frozen	10 puffs	175	3	8	24	2.5

	Portion	Calories (kcal)	Protein (g)	Total Fat (g)	Carbo-hydrate (g)	Total Dietary Fiber (g)
Potato salad, home prepared	1 cup	358	7	21	28	3.3
Scalloped						
From dry mix, with whole milk, butter	1 cup	228	5	11	31	2.7
From home recipe, with butter	1 cup	211	7	9	26	4.7
Pumpkin						
Cooked, mashed	1 cup	49	2	Tr	12	2.7
Canned	1 cup	83	3	1	20	7.1
Radishes, raw (¾"–1" dia.)	1 radish	1	Tr	Tr	Tr	0.1
Rutabagas, cooked, drained, cubes	1 cup	66	2	Tr	15	3.1
Sauerkraut, canned, solids and liquid	1 cup	45	2	Tr	10	5.9
Seaweed						
Kelp, raw	2 TB.	4	Tr	Tr	1	0.1
Spirulina, dried	1 TB.	3	1	Tr	Tr	Tr
Shallots, raw, chopped	1 TB.	7	Tr	Tr	2	0.2
Soybeans, green, cooked, drained	1 cup	254	22	12	20	7.6
Spinach						
Raw						
Chopped	1 cup	7	1	Tr	1	0.8
Leaf	1 leaf	2	Tr	Tr	Tr	0.3
Cooked, drained						
From raw	1 cup	41	5	Tr	7	4.3
From frozen (chopped or leaf)	1 cup	53	6	Tr	10	5.7
Canned, drained	1 cup	49	6	1	7	5.1
Squash						
Summer (all varieties), sliced						
Raw	1 cup	23	1	Tr	5	2.1
Cooked, drained	1 cup	36	2	1	8	2.5
Winter (all varieties), baked, cubes	1 cup	80	2	1	18	5.7
Winter, butternut, frozen, cooked, mashed	1 cup	94	3	Tr	24	2.2

	Portion	Calories (kcal)	Protein (g)	Total Fat (g)	Carbo-hydrate (g)	Total Dietary Fiber (g)
Sweet potatoes						
Cooked (2" dia., 5" long raw)						
Baked, with skin	1 potato	150	3	Tr	35	4.4
Boiled, without skin	1 potato	164	3	Tr	38	2.8
Candied (2½" × 2" piece)	1 piece	144	1	3	29	2.5
Canned						
Syrup pack, drained	1 cup	212	3	1	50	5.9
Vacuum pack, mashed	1 cup	232	4	1	54	4.6
Tomatillos, raw	1 medium	11	Tr	Tr	2	0.6
Tomatoes						
Raw, year-round average						
Chopped or sliced	1 cup	38	2	1	8	2.0
Slice, medium, ¼" thick	1 slice	4	Tr	Tr	1	0.2
Whole						
Cherry	1 cherry	4	Tr	Tr	1	0.2
Medium, 2⅗" dia.	1 tomato	26	1	Tr	6	1.4
Canned, solids and liquid	1 cup	46	2	Tr	10	2.4
Sun dried						
Plain	1 piece	5	Tr	Tr	1	0.2
Packed in oil, drained	1 piece	6	Tr	Tr	1	0.2
Tomato juice, canned, with salt added	1 cup	41	2	Tr	10	1.0
Tomato products, canned						
Paste	1 cup	215	10	1	51	10.7
Puree	1 cup	100	4	Tr	24	5.0
Sauce	1 cup	74	3	Tr	18	3.4
Spaghetti/marinara/pasta sauce (see Soups, sauces, and gravies)						
Stewed	1 cup	71	2	Tr	17	2.6

	Portion	Calories (kcal)	Protein (g)	Total Fat (g)	Carbo-hydrate (g)	Total Dietary Fiber (g)
Turnips, cooked, cubes	1 cup	33	1	Tr	8	3.1
Turnip greens, cooked, drained						
From raw (leaves and stems)	1 cup	29	2	Tr	6	5.0
From frozen (chopped)	1 cup	49	5	1	8	5.6
Vegetable juice cocktail, canned	1 cup	46	2	Tr	11	1.9
Vegetables, mixed						
Canned, drained	1 cup	77	4	Tr	15	4.9
Frozen, cooked, drained	1 cup	107	5	Tr	24	8.0
Water chestnuts, canned, slices, solids and liquids	1 cup	70	1	Tr	17	3.5

Miscellaneous Items

	Portion	Calories (kcal)	Protein (g)	Total Fat (g)	Carbo-hydrate (g)	Total Dietary Fiber (g)
Bacon bits, meatless	1 TB.	31	2	2	2	0.7
Baking powders for home use						
Double acting						
Sodium aluminum sulfate	1 tsp.	2	0	0	1	Tr
Straight phosphate	1 tsp.	2	Tr	0	1	Tr
Low sodium	1 tsp.	5	Tr	Tr	2	0.1
Baking soda	1 tsp.	0	0	0	0	0.0
Beef jerky	1 large piece	81	7	5	2	0.4
Catsup	1 cup	250	4	1	65	3.1
	1 TB.	16	Tr	Tr	4	0.2
	1 packet	6	Tr	Tr	2	0.1
Celery seed	1 tsp.	8	Tr	1	1	0.2
Chili powder	1 tsp.	8	Tr	Tr	1	
Chocolate, unsweetened, baking						
Solid	1 square	148	3	16	8	4.4
Liquid	1 oz.	134	3	14	10	5.1
Cinnamon	1 tsp.	6	Tr	Tr	2	1.2
Cocoa powder, unsweetened	1 cup	197	17	12	47	28.6
	1 TB.	12	1	1	3	1.8

	Portion	Calories (kcal)	Protein (g)	Total Fat (g)	Carbo-hydrate (g)	Total Dietary Fiber (g)
Cream of tartar	1 tsp.	8	0	0	2	Tr
Curry powder	1 tsp.	7	Tr	Tr	1	0.7
Garlic powder	1 tsp.	9	Tr	Tr	2	0.3
Horseradish, prepared	1 tsp.	2	Tr	Tr	1	0.2
Mustard, prepared, yellow	1 tsp. or 1 packet	3	Tr	Tr	Tr	0.2
Olives, canned						
Pickled, green	5 medium	20	Tr	2	Tr	0.2
Ripe, black	5 large	25	Tr	2	1	0.7
Onion powder	1 tsp.	7	Tr	Tr	2	0.1
Oregano, ground	1 tsp.	5	Tr	Tr	1	0.6
Paprika	1 tsp.	6	Tr	Tr	1	0.4
Parsley, dried	1 TB.	4	Tr	Tr	1	0.4
Pepper, black	1 tsp.	5	Tr	Tr	1	0.6
Pickles, cucumber						
Dill, whole, medium (3¾" long)	1 pickle	12	Tr	Tr	3	0.8
Fresh (bread and butter pickles), slices 1½" dia., ¼" thick	3 slices	18	Tr	Tr	4	0.4
Pickle relish, sweet	1 TB.	20	Tr	Tr	5	0.2
Pork skins/rinds, plain	1 oz.	155	17	9	0	0.0
Potato chips						
Regular						
Plain						
Salted	1 oz.	152	2	10	15	1.3
Unsalted	1 oz.	152	2	10	15	1.4
Barbecue flavor	1 oz.	139	2	9	15	1.2
Sour cream and onion flavor	1 oz.	151	2	10	15	1.5
Reduced fat	1 oz.	134	2	6	19	1.7
Fat free, made with olestra	1 oz.	75	2	Tr	17	1.1
Made from dried potatoes						
Plain	1 oz.	158	2	11	14	1.0
Sour cream and onion flavor	1 oz.	155	2	10	15	0.3

	Portion	Calories (kcal)	Protein (g)	Total Fat (g)	Carbo-hydrate (g)	Total Dietary Fiber (g)
Reduced fat	1 oz.	142	2	7	18	1.0
Salt	1 tsp.	0	0	0	0	0.0
Trail mix						
Regular, with raisins, chocolate chips, salted nuts, and seeds	1 cup	707	21	47	66	8.8
Tropical	1 cup	570	9	24	92	10.6
Vanilla extract	1 tsp.	12	Tr	Tr	1	0.0
Vinegar						
Cider	1 TB.	2	0	0	1	0.0
Distilled	1 TB.	2	0	0	1	0.0
Yeast, baker's						
Dry, active	1 package	21	3	Tr	3	1.5
	1 tsp.	12	2	Tr	2	0.8
Compressed	1 cake	18	1	Tr	3	1.4

Online Resources

Nobody goes it alone, especially when you're deep in the throes of a diet; particularly a diet that might have many rules to follow, an exacting ratio of nutrients, and other must-remember facts buzzing through your head. Well, sweat this no more. The following are a handful of sites dedicated to making your dieting life much, much easier.

The U.S. Department of Agriculture's Nutrient Data Laboratory
www.nal.usda.gov/fnic/foodcomp/Data/SR16-1/wtrank/wt_rank.html

This site shows your tax dollars at work—and how! At this site you can click on any of 38 food nutrient categories that include vitamins, minerals, fats, and more and find out how much is in the food you eat. It will even tell you how much water is in your food. This site spits out an Adobe Acrobat report that lists hundreds of foods sorted either alphabetically or by specific nutrient. The reports are adapted from the 2002 revision of *Home and Garden* Bulletin No. 72, Nutritive Value of Foods.

The Friedman School of Nutrition Science and Policy at Tufts University
nutrition.tufts.edu

This site is one of the best, most scientifically sound, and most balanced nutrition sites you will run across. Rummage around; there are plenty of stories and reports, and you might be surprised at what the latest research shows about the foods you eat.

Interactive Healthy Eating Index
147.208.9.133/Default.asp

Don't pay money to get a computer program to add up all your food and give you detailed nutrient values. This site from those wonderful folks at the U.S. Department of Agriculture's Center for Nutrition Policy and Promotion do it all for you. And it's all free. A tiny little login will get you to the food intake area where you search an extensive list of foods and choose what you've eaten, are about to eat, or only wish you could eat. Click the Analyze button, and you'll see a detailed report on the nutrient intake based on your quantity. Eating more? Just keep adding foods, and it'll keep track of everything.

Physical Activity Evaluator
147.208.9.133/Default.asp

We bet you didn't know that doing 20 minutes of the hula will burn off 98 calories. We didn't either until we explored this very extensive exercise flavor of the Interactive Healthy Eating Index. Same drill as above to get in, but just click the Proceed to Physical Activity link after you successfully log into the site. It will even keep a history of your physical activity and generate a graph that plots it. It also generates a report that tells you if your exercising needs improvement. Everyone's a critic.

Interactive Menu Planner
hin.nhlbi.nih.gov/menuplanner/menu.cgi

The National Heart, Lung, and Blood Institute has come up with this nifty menu planner that figures all the carbs, calories, and fat for you. Pick common foods from drop-down menus on the right side, enter how many servings you want, and the planner automatically comes up with all the numbers on the left side. The slant tips toward counting calories, but it's a great tool for low-carb dieters, also. The best part: It keeps track of your meal selections on a daily menu below the interactive part. It's great for printing out and taking along to the grocery store.

Low-Carb Internet Groups
www.lowcarbsuccess.net/links.htm

This is part of author Laura Richard's website that promotes her excellent book, *The Secret to Low Carb Success!* Here you'll find lists and descriptions of a myriad of sites, at least one of which will be good for you. The sites run the gamut from discussion groups about the Atkins diet to general groups and sites that offer everything from chat rooms and bulletin boards to recipes and inspirational success stories.

Glossary

aerobic   Means "with oxygen," but when it comes to exercise, it means doing an activity for at least 15 minutes, using major muscles at a pace that is at least 65 percent of your maximum heart rate.

anabolic steroids   Man-made chemicals that mimic the effects of male sex hormones. Bodybuilders and athletes often use them to increase muscle mass. Reported side effects include irritability and aggression.

anaerobic   Means "without oxygen." This refers to exercise done by muscles at a high intensity for a short period of time.

apnea   A frequent disruption in sleep from blocked or constricted airflow caused by a physical obstruction in the upper airway or a missed signal from the brain to the respiratory muscles. It affects about 2.5 million of the 30 million Americans who snore.

Body Mass Index (BMI)   A relationship between weight and height that is a measure of fat in the body. It is figured by dividing your weight in pounds by the square of your height in inches and then multiplying that number by 703.

corticosteroid   A type of hormone made naturally by the adrenal glands. Its many functions include regulating fluids and minerals, the metabolism, growth, body temperature, and much more. When man-made, the drug treats inflammation and allergies and dampens immune response, among other uses.

cortisol   A hormone made by the adrenal glands; it is important in activating the immune system and processing carbohydrates. High amounts of it are released in moments of stress.

diastolic   The bottom of the two blood pressure numbers. It reflects the blood's pressure when the heart is at rest between beats.

diuretic   A substance that tends to increase the amount of urine passed by the body.

ephedrine   The main active ingredient in ephedra (also called Ma huang), a naturally occurring substance that comes from plants. Ephedra is a stimulant that acts like adrenaline and may have dangerous effects on the heart and blood pressure.

French paradox   The contradiction between the idea that the French diet, while much higher in saturated fat than an American diet, may cause fewer cancers and less death from heart disease. Many studies say this is because the French drink more wine than we do.

glucose   The main source of your body's energy; it is made from carbohydrates in food and transported through the body in the bloodstream.

glycogen   The stored form of glucose in the liver and muscles. It's produced when blood sugar levels are high.

hypertension   When your blood goes through your vessels with a force greater than normal. The pressure from this force can strain your heart and injure your arteries.

ligaments   Cord-like tissues that connect bones to other bones or to cartilage. They stabilize joints.

lipids   Fatty substances in the blood that are sources of fuel and are easily stored by the body.

metabolism   Everything your body does, chemically and physically, to keep growing and working. This has to do with the breaking down and building up of complex substances in the body. Breaking them down releases energy so that other complex substances, such as tissue and muscles, can be created.

monosodium glutamate (MSG)   Used as a flavor enhancer. In the last three decades, people have reported such reactions to it as worsened asthma and headaches.

monounsaturated fat   Found in high concentrations in some oils, such as olive oil, canola oil, and peanut oil. It is linked to raising levels of "good" cholesterol and lowering levels of "bad" cholesterol.

nitrites   Chemicals used to enhance color and flavor; they are also used as preservatives, mainly to prevent botulism.

polyunsaturated fat   Contained in many vegetable oils such as corn, soybean, and sunflower, in nuts, and in high-fat fish, such as tuna.

saturated fats   Generally solid at room temperature, they most often come from animal sources—although palm and coconut oils are also high in this fat. This type of fat is considered one of the least healthy and is linked to raising blood cholesterol levels.

serotonin   A brain chemical that is key in regulating mood, appetite, sleep, body temperature, blood pressure, heart beat, and other functions.

systolic   The top of the two numbers that measure blood pressure. This reflects the highest blood pressure reached as the blood is pumped out of the heart.

trans-fatty acids   Made when liquid oils are combined with hydrogen and heated to form solid fats, such as shortening. They're considered the least healthy of all the fats.

Index